PN Mental Health Nursing
REVIEW MODULE EDITION 12.0

Contributors

Alissa Althoff, Ed.D, MSN, RN

Mendy Gearhart, DNP, MSN, CCCE

Norma Jean Henry, MSN/Ed, RN

Honey C. Holman, MSN, RN

Janean Johnson, DNP, RN, CNE

Beth Cusatis Phillips, PhD, RN, CNE, CHSE

Pamela Roland, MSN, MBA, RN

Consultants

Brandon Dominguez, DNP, RN, CHSE

Lynne M. Kuhl, MSN/Ed, BA, RN

INTELLECTUAL PROPERTY NOTICE

Director of content review: Kristen Lawler

Director of development: Derek Prater

Project management: Meri Ann Mason

Coordination of content review: Alissa Althoff, Honey C. Holman

Copy editing: Kelly Von Lunen, Tricia Lunt, Bethany Robertson, Kya Rodgers, Rebecca Her, Sam Shiel, Alethea Surland, Graphic World

Layout: Bethany Robertson, Maureen Bradshaw, Haylee Hedge, scottie. o

Illustrations: Randi Hardy, Graphic World

Online media: Brant Stacy, Ron Hanson, Britney Frerking, Trevor Lund

Interior book design: Spring Lenox

IMPORTANT NOTICE TO THE READER

User's Guide

Welcome to the Assessment Technologies Institute® PN Mental Health Nursing Review Module Edition 12.0. The mission of ATI's Content Mastery Series® Review Modules is to provide user-friendly compendiums of nursing knowledge that will:
- Help you locate important information quickly.
- Assist in your learning efforts.
- Provide exercises for applying your nursing knowledge.
- Facilitate your entry into the nursing profession as a newly licensed nurse.

ORGANIZATION

This Review Module is organized into units covering foundations for mental health nursing, traditional nonpharmacological therapies, psychobiologic disorders, specific populations, and critical mental health concerns. Chapters within these units conform to one of four organizing principles for presenting the content.
- Nursing concepts
- Procedures
- Disorders

Nursing concepts chapters begin with an overview describing the central concept and its relevance to nursing. Subordinate themes are covered in outline form to demonstrate relationships and present the information in a clear, succinct manner.

Procedures chapters include an overview describing the procedure(s) covered in the chapter. These chapters provide nursing knowledge relevant to each procedure, including indications, nursing considerations, and complications.

Disorders chapters include an overview describing the disorder. These chapters cover assessments, including risk factors and expected findings, and patient-centered care, including nursing care, medications, therapeutic procedures, and interprofessional care.

ACTIVE LEARNING SCENARIOS AND APPLICATION EXERCISES

Each chapter includes opportunities for you to test your knowledge and to practice applying that knowledge. Active Learning Scenario exercises pose a nursing scenario and then direct you to use an ATI Active Learning Template (included at the back of this book) to record the important knowledge a nurse should apply to the scenario. An example is then provided to which you can compare your completed Active Learning Template. The Application Exercises include NCLEX-style questions, such as multiple-choice and multiple-select items, providing you with opportunities to practice answering the kinds of questions you might expect to see on ATI assessments or the NCLEX. After the Application Exercises, an answer key is provided, along with rationales.

NCLEX® CONNECTIONS

To prepare for the NCLEX-PN, it is important to understand how the content in this Review Module is connected to the NCLEX-PN test plan. You can find information on the detailed test plan at the National Council of State Boards of Nursing's website, www.ncsbn.org. When reviewing content in this Review Module, regularly ask yourself, "How does this content fit into the test plan, and what types of questions related to this content should I expect?"

To help you in this process, we've included NCLEX Connections at the beginning of each unit and with each question in the Application Exercises Answer Keys. The NCLEX Connections at the beginning of each unit point out areas of the detailed test plan that relate to the content within that unit. The NCLEX Connections attached to the Application Exercises Answer Keys demonstrate how each exercise fits within the detailed content outline. These NCLEX Connections will help you understand how the detailed content outline is organized, starting with major client needs categories and subcategories and followed by related content areas and tasks. The major client needs categories are:
- Safe and Effective Care Environment
  - Management of Care
  - Safety and Infection Control
- Health Promotion and Maintenance
- Psychosocial Integrity
- Physiological Integrity
  - Basic Care and Comfort
  - Pharmacological and Parenteral Therapies
  - Reduction of Risk Potential
  - Physiological Adaptation

An NCLEX Connection might, for example, alert you that content within a unit is related to:
- Psychosocial Integrity
  - Behavioral Interventions
    - Incorporate behavioral management techniques when caring for a client.

QSEN COMPETENCIES

As you use the Review Modules, you will note the integration of the Quality and Safety Education for Nurses (QSEN) competencies throughout the chapters. These competencies are integral components of the curriculum of many nursing programs in the United States and prepare you to provide safe, high-quality care as a newly licensed nurse. Icons appear to draw your attention to the six QSEN competencies.

Safety: The minimization of risk factors that could cause injury or harm while promoting quality care and maintaining a secure environment for clients, self, and others.

Patient-Centered Care: The provision of caring and compassionate, culturally sensitive care that addresses clients' physiological, psychological, sociological, spiritual, and cultural needs, preferences, and values.

Evidence-Based Practice: The use of current knowledge from research and other credible sources, on which to base clinical judgment and client care.

Informatics: The use of information technology as a communication and information-gathering tool that supports clinical decision-making and scientifically based nursing practice.

Quality Improvement: Care related and organizational processes that involve the development and implementation of a plan to improve health care services and better meet clients' needs.

Teamwork and Collaboration: The delivery of client care in partnership with multidisciplinary members of the health care team to achieve continuity of care and positive client outcomes.

ICONS

Icons are used throughout the Review Module to draw your attention to particular areas. Keep an eye out for these icons.

(N) This icon is used for NCLEX Connections.

(G) This icon indicates gerontological considerations, or knowledge specific to the care of older adult clients.

Qs This icon is used for content related to safety and is a QSEN competency. When you see this icon, take note of safety concerns or steps that nurses can take to ensure client safety and a safe environment.

QPCC This icon is a QSEN competency that indicates the importance of a holistic approach to providing care.

QEBP This icon, a QSEN competency, points out the integration of research into clinical practice.

QI This icon is a QSEN competency and highlights the use of information technology to support nursing practice.

QQI This icon is used to focus on the QSEN competency of integrating planning processes to meet clients' needs.

QTC This icon highlights the QSEN competency of care delivery using an interprofessional approach.

SDoH This icon highlights content related to social determinants of health.

M◇ This icon appears at the top-right of pages and indicates availability of an online media supplement, such as a graphic, animation, or video. If you have an electronic copy of the Review Module, this icon will appear alongside clickable links to media supplements. If you have a hard copy version of the Review Module, visit www.atitesting.com for details on how to access these features.

FEEDBACK

ATI welcomes feedback regarding this Review Module. Please provide comments to comments@atitesting.com.

As needed updates to the Review Modules are identified, changes to the text are made for subsequent printings of the book and for subsequent releases of the electronic version. For the printed books, print runs are based on when existing stock is depleted. For the electronic versions, a number of factors influence the update schedule. As such, ATI encourages faculty and students to refer to the Review Module addendums for information on what updates have been made. These addendums, which are available in the Help/FAQs on the student site and the Resources/eBooks & Active Learning on the faculty site, are updated regularly and always include the most current information on updates to the Review Modules.

Table of Contents

NCLEX® Connections

When reviewing the following chapters, keep in mind the relevant topics and tasks of the NCLEX outline.

Coordinated Care

ADVOCACY: Advocate for client rights and needs.

CLIENT RIGHTS: Recognize client right to refuse treatment/procedures.

CONFIDENTIALITY/INFORMATION SECURITY: Maintain client confidentiality.

ETHICAL PRACTICE: Practice in a manner consistent with code of ethics for nurses.

LEGAL RESPONSIBILITIES
Identify legal issues affecting staff and client.

Follow regulation/policy for reporting specific issues.

Safety and Infection Control

ACCIDENT/ERROR/INJURY PREVENTION: Protect client from accident/error/injury.

LEAST RESTRICTIVE RESTRAINTS AND SAFETY DEVICES:
Implement least restrictive restraints or seclusion.

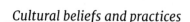
UNIT 1   FOUNDATIONS FOR MENTAL HEALTH NURSING

CHAPTER 1 # Basic Mental Health Nursing Concepts

Provision of care to clients in mental health settings is based on standards of care set by the American Nurses Association, the American Psychiatric Nurses Association, and the International Society of Psychiatric-Mental Health Nurses.

Nurses working in mental health settings should use the nursing process, as well as a holistic approach (biological, social, psychological, and spiritual aspects) to care for clients.

Nurses should use various methods to collect data from clients. These methods include observation, interviewing, physical examination, and collaboration.

DATA COLLECTION

- Perform physical data collection as indicated for client condition or policy.
  - Use touch to communicate caring as appropriate. However, respect the client's personal space if they do not wish to be touched.
  - Be sure to include questions relating to difficulty sleeping, incontinence, falls or other injuries, depression, dizziness, and loss of energy.
  - Include the family and significant others as appropriate.
  - Obtain a detailed medication history.
  - Following the interview, summarize and ask for feedback from the client.
- Each encounter with a client involves an ongoing data collection.

PSYCHOSOCIAL HISTORY

- Determine the client's perception of own health, beliefs about illness and wellness. Qpcc
- Activity/leisure activities, how the client passes time.
- Determine the client's use of substances and any history of a substance use disorder.
- Determine the client's stress level and coping abilities: usual coping strategies, support systems.

Cultural beliefs and practices

- Identify the client's culture, express interest in the client's culture, and integrate it as best as possible into the client's plan of care.
- Determine cultural factors that can impact the client's care.

  > For example: Does the client's diet consist of culture-specific foods? Does the client have specific beliefs or practices regarding health care? How is the client's diagnosis viewed in their culture?

- The nurse's awareness of culture alleviates stereotyping and stigmatizing.
- Use a trained interpreter when needed.

Spiritual and religious beliefs

Spiritual and religious beliefs affect the way in which a client finds meaning, hope, purpose, and a sense of peace.
- Spirituality refers to a client's internal values, sense of morality, and how the client views the purpose of life. The client might not connect these spiritual views with religion.
- Religion refers to a client's beliefs according to an organized set of patterns of worship and rituals.
- Determine the client's support systems and assist the client to identify support persons and resources.
- Assist in locating a spiritual or religious leader if needed.

MENTAL STATUS EXAMINATION (MSE)

Level of consciousness

The level of consciousness is described using the following terms. Observed behaviors are included in the documentation.

Alert: The client is responsive and able to fully respond by opening their eyes and responding to a normal tone of voice and speech. The client answers questions spontaneously and appropriately.

Lethargic: The client is able to open their eyes and respond but is drowsy and falls asleep readily.

Stuporous: The client requires vigorous or painful stimuli (pinching a tendon or rubbing the sternum) to elicit a brief response. The client might not be able to respond verbally.

Comatose: The client is unconscious and does not respond to painful stimuli.
- Abnormal posturing in the client who is comatose
  - **Decorticate rigidity**: Flexion and internal rotation of upper-extremity joints and legs
  - **Decerebrate rigidity**: Neck and elbow extension, wrist and finger flexion

Physical appearance

Examination includes data collection of personal hygiene, grooming, nutritional status, clothing choice, and whether the client looks older than their stated age. Expected findings with regard to this data are that the client is well-kempt, clean, and dressed appropriately for the given environment.

Behavior

Examination includes data collection of voluntary and involuntary body movements, and eye contact.

Mood: A client's mood provides information about the emotion that the client is feeling.

Affect: A client's affect is an objective expression of mood (a flat affect or a lack of facial expression).

Cognitive and intellectual abilities

- Determine the client's orientation to time, person, and place.
- Check the client's memory, both recent and remote.
  - **Immediate**: Ask the client to repeat a series of numbers or a list of objects.
  - **Recent**: Ask the client to recall recent events (visitors from the current day) or the purpose of the current mental health appointment or admission.
  - **Remote**: Ask the client to state a fact from their past that is verifiable (their birth date or their mother's maiden name).
- Identify the client's level of knowledge. For example, ask the client what they know about their current illness or hospitalization.
- Check the client's ability to calculate. For example, can the client count backward from 100 in serials of 7?
- Determine the client's ability to think abstractly. For example, can the client explain the similarities between two objects? ("How are cars and trains similar?") The ability to explain this demonstrates a higher-level thought process. Be sensitive to cultural or primary language differences.
- Perform objective data collection of the client's perception of his illness.
- Determine the client's judgment based on the client's answer to a hypothetical question. For example, how would they answer the question, "What would you do if there were a fire in your room?" The client should provide a logical response.
- Check the client's rate and volume of speech, as well as the quality of their language. The client's speech and responses should be meaningful, articulate, and appropriate.

STANDARDIZED SCREENING TOOLS

There are a number of standardized rating scales that can be used for evaluation and monitoring of clients.

Adverse Childhood Experiences Questionnaire

Brief Patient Health Questionnaire (Brief PHQ)

Mini-mental state examination (MMSE): This examination is used to objectively collect data about a client's cognitive status by evaluating the following. Q EBP
- Orientation to time and place
- Attention span and ability to calculate by counting backward by seven
- Registration and recalling of objects
- Language, including naming of objects, following of commands, and ability to write

Pain data collection tools: Pain rating tools include visual analogue scales, Wong-Baker FACES Pain Rating Scale, the Faces Pain Scale-Revised, the McGill Pain Questionnaire (MPQ), and the Pain Assessment in Advanced Dementia (PAINAD) scale.

CONSIDERATIONS ACROSS THE LIFESPAN

Children and adolescents

Data collection includes temperament, social and environmental factors, cultural and religious concerns, and developmental level. The client should be the source of the information but with children and adolescents; caregivers can also provide valuable information. Q PCC
- Mentally healthy children and adolescents trust others, view the world as safe, accurately interpret their environments, master developmental tasks, and use appropriate coping skills.
- Children and adolescents experience some of the same mental health problems as adults.
- Mental health and developmental disorders are not always easily diagnosed, potentially resulting in delayed or inadequate treatment interventions. Factors contributing to this include the following.
  - Lack of the ability or necessary skills to describe what is happening
  - A wide variation of "normal" behavior, especially in different developmental stages
- Check for mood; anxiety; developmental, behavioral, and eating disorders; and risk for self-injury or suicide.
- Use the HEADSSS standardized data collection tool: Q EBP
  - **Home environment:** What is the client's relationship like with their guardians and other family members living in the home?
  - **Education/employment**: Is the client employed? How is the client's school performance?
  - **Activities:** Does the client participate in sports or other activities? How does the client interact with peers?
  - **Drug and substance use:** Does the client use substances (alcohol, tobacco, or illicit drugs)?
  - **Sexuality:** Has the client engaged in any sexual activity or had any sexual encounters?
  - **Suicide/depression**: Is the client at risk for suicide or self-injury? Does the client have indications of depression?
  - **Safety**: Is the client exposed to abuse in the home or violence in the neighborhood?

Older adults

- In addition to the aforementioned data collection, a comprehensive evaluation of the older adult client includes the following.
  - Functional ability (the ability to independently get dressed or manage household tasks)
  - Economic and social status
  - Environmental factors (stairways in the home) that can affect the client's well-being and lifestyle

- Standardized data collection tools that are appropriate for the older adult population include the following.
  - Geriatric Depression Scale (short form) ⊙
  - Michigan Alcoholism Screening Test: Geriatric Version
  - MMSE
- Conduct an interview of all clients in the following manner.
  - Use a private, quiet space with adequate lighting to accommodate for impaired vision and hearing.
  - Make an introduction, and determine the client's name and pronoun preference.
  - Stand or sit at the client's level to conduct the interview, rather than standing over a client who is lying in bed or sitting in a chair.

Social determinants of mental health

Social determinants of mental health (SDoMH) are the ways clients live and work and how this shapes their health outcomes. These can be rooted in health inequalities. Disparities in mental health care, treatment, and accessibility profoundly influence the outcomes and experiences of clients. Understanding disparities in mental health care requires consideration of the SDoMH, which have been identified by the World Health Organization. Although not fundamentally different from the social determinates of health (SDOH) as they are linked to health, mental health experts understand that the solutions for mental health may require a different approach.

TRAUMA INFORMED CARE

Nurses are sensitive to the importance of screening for interpersonal violence and trauma to better understand current client behaviors and relationships.
- Realize that trauma can affect people and groups
- Recognize the signs of trauma
- Organized responses to trauma
- Resisting re-traumatization

MENTAL HEALTH DIAGNOSES

- The *Diagnostic and Statistical Manual of Mental Disorders, 5th Edition, Text Revision* (DSM-5-TR), published by the American Psychiatric Association, is used by mental health professionals to diagnose mental health disorders in clients following standard criteria. It includes expected data collection findings for disorders and helps with planning, implementing, and evaluating care.
- Nurses use diagnoses from the North American Nursing Diagnosis Association (NANDA) to provide the basis of appropriate nursing interventions for clients. ○EBP

SERIOUS MENTAL ILLNESS
- Includes disorders classified as severe and persistent mental illnesses
- Clients often have difficulty with activities of daily living (ADLs)
- Are lifelong disorders that can have remissions and exacerbations

ROLE AND LIFE CHANGES

- Role transitions include loss of employment, divorce, retirement, grand-parenthood, widowhood, death of guardian, and becoming a caregiver or recipient of care.
- Some role changes are predicted (an upcoming retirement). However, the client might find that others are unexpected (becoming the recipient of care due to a sudden illness or injury).
- Identifying the client's ability to adapt and cope includes the following.
  - Health status and functional abilities
  - Living arrangements and employability
  - Personality factors, such as attitudes
  - Client, caregiver and family observations
  - Levels of information, such as community programs
  - Medication use and supplemental services
- Evaluating whether client has successfully adapted includes the following.
  - Able to state positive coping behaviors
  - Able to identify maladaptive coping behaviors
  - Able to participate in community resources
  - Able to list stress reduction techniques
  - Able to maintain housing and employment

THERAPEUTIC STRATEGIES IN THE MENTAL HEALTH SETTING

Counseling
- Using therapeutic communication skills
- Assisting with problem solving
- Crisis intervention
- Stress management

Milieu therapy
- Orienting the client to the physical setting
- Identifying rules and boundaries of the setting
- Ensuring a safe environment for the client
- Assisting the client to participate in appropriate activities

Screening
- Trauma history
- Risk for suicide and non-suicidal self-injury
- Substance use
- Coping skills
- Support systems

Promotion of self-care activities
- Offering assistance with self-care tasks
- Allowing time for the client to complete self-care tasks
- Setting incentives to promote client self-care

Psychobiological interventions
- Administering prescribed medications
- Reinforcing teaching to the client/family about medications
- Monitoring for adverse effects and effectiveness of pharmacological therapy

Cognitive and behavioral therapies
- Modeling
- Operant conditioning
- Systematic desensitization

Health teaching: Reinforcing teaching social and coping skills, as well as stress reduction techniques.

Health promotion and health maintenance
- Assisting the client with cessation of smoking
- Monitoring other health conditions

Case management: Coordinating holistic care to include medical, mental health, and social services

Active Learning Scenario

A nurse is assisting with the admission of an older adult client who has depression to an acute mental health facility. Use the ATI Active Learning Template: Basic Concept to complete this item.

UNDERLYING PRINCIPLES
- Identify the standardized data collection tool the nurse should use to identify the older adult client's severity of depression.
- Identify at least four data collection/communication techniques the nurse should use when collecting data on the older adult client.

NURSING INTERVENTIONS: Identify at least three factors the nurse should collect data from to determine if role and life changes are contributing to the client's depression.

Application Exercises

1. A nurse in an outpatient mental health clinic is preparing to assist with conducting an initial client interview. When conducting the interview, which of the following actions should the nurse identify as the priority?
   - A. Coordinate holistic care with social services.
   - B. Identify the client's perception of their mental health status.
   - C. Include the client's family in the interview.
   - D. Teach the client about their current mental health disorder.

2. A charge nurse is discussing mental status examinations with a newly licensed nurse. Which of the following statements by the newly licensed nurse indicates an understanding of the teaching? (Select all that apply.)
   - A. "To assess cognitive ability, I should ask the client to count backward by sevens."
   - B. "To assess affect, I should observe the client's facial expression."
   - C. "To assess language ability, I should instruct the client to write a sentence."
   - D. "To assess remote memory, I should have the client repeat a list of objects."
   - E. "To assess the client's abstract thinking, I should ask the client to identify our most recent presidents."

3. A nurse is assisting with a peer group discussion about the *Diagnostic and Statistical Manual of Mental Disorders, 5th Edition Text Revision* (DSM-5-TR). Which of the following information should the nurse include in the discussion? (Select all that apply.)
   - A. The DSM-5-TR includes client education handouts for mental health disorders.
   - B. The DSM-5-TR establishes diagnostic criteria for individual mental health disorders.
   - C. The DSM-5-TR indicates recommended pharmacological treatment for mental health disorders.
   - D. The DSM-5-TR assists nurses in planning care for clients who have mental health disorders.
   - E. The DSM-5-TR indicates expected data collection findings of mental health disorders.

4. A nurse is assisting with the plan of care for a client who has a mental health disorder. Which of the following actions should the nurse include as a psychobiological intervention?
   - A. Assist the client with systematic desensitization therapy.
   - B. Teach the client appropriate coping mechanisms.
   - C. Assess the client for comorbid health conditions.
   - D. Monitor the client for adverse effects of medications.

Application Exercises Key

1. B. **CORRECT:** The first action the nurse should take when using the nursing process is collecting data, identifying the client's perception of their mental health status provides important information about the client's psychosocial history. The nurse should coordinate holistic care for the client with social services as part of case management. However, another action is the priority. If the client wishes, it is appropriate to include the client's family in the interview. However, another action is the priority. It is appropriate to teach the client about their disorder. However, another action is the priority.

   Ⓝ *NCLEX® Connection: Health Promotion and Maintenance, Data Collection Techniques*

2. A, B, C. **CORRECT:** When evaluating a newly licensed nurse's understanding of mental status examinations counting backward by sevens is an appropriate technique to assess a client's cognitive ability, observing a client's facial expressions is appropriate when assessing affect, writing a sentence is an indication of language ability. These statements all indicate an understanding of mental status examinations. Asking the client to repeat a list of objects is appropriate to assess immediate, rather than remote memory. Asking the client to identify recent presidents is appropriate to assess cognitive knowledge rather than abstract thinking.

   Ⓝ *NCLEX® Connection: Psychosocial Integrity, Mental Health Concepts*

3. B, D, E. **CORRECT:** The DSM-5-TR establishes diagnostic criteria for mental health disorders. Nurses use the DSM-5-TR to plan, implement, and evaluate care for client's who have mental health disorders. The DSM-5-TR identifies expected findings for mental health disorders.

   Ⓝ *NCLEX® Connection: Psychosocial Integrity, Mental Health Concepts*

4. D. **CORRECT:** When generating solutions for a client who has a mental health disorder the nurse should include the following psychobiological intervention, monitoring for adverse effects of medications. Assisting with systematic desensitization therapy is a cognitive and behavioral intervention. Teaching appropriate coping mechanisms is a counseling or health teaching intervention. Assessing for comorbid health conditions is health promotion and maintenance, rather than a psychobiological intervention.

   Ⓝ *NCLEX® Connection: Psychosocial Integrity, Mental Health Concepts*

Active Learning Scenario Key

Using the ATI Active Learning Template: Basic Concept

UNDERLYING PRINCIPLES
- Standardized data collection tool for depression: Geriatric Depression Scale
- Data collection/communication techniques
  - Use a private, quiet space with adequate lighting to accommodate for impaired vision and hearing.
  - Make an introduction, and determine the client's name preference.
  - Stand or sit at the client's level to conduct the interview.
  - Use touch to communicate caring as appropriate.
  - Include questions relating to difficulty sleeping, incontinence, falls or other injuries, depression, dizziness, and loss of energy.
  - Include the family and significant others as appropriate.
  - Assist with collecting data about medication history.
  - Following the interview, summarize and ask for feedback from the client.

NURSING INTERVENTIONS: Identify role and life changes
- Recent role transitions and whether they were expected or unexpected
- Client's knowledge and use of positive coping behaviors
- Participation in community resources
- Client's knowledge and use of stress reduction techniques
- Ability to maintain housing or employment

Ⓝ *NCLEX® Connection: Psychosocial Integrity, Mental Health Concepts*

CHAPTER 2

CHAPTER 2 *Legal and Ethical Issues*

A nurse who works in the mental health setting is responsible for practicing ethically, competently, safely, and in a manner consistent with all local, state, and federal laws.

Nurses must have an understanding of ethical principles and how they apply when providing care for clients in mental health settings.

Nurses are responsible for understanding and protecting client rights.

LEGAL RIGHTS OF CLIENTS IN THE MENTAL HEALTH SETTING

- Clients who have a mental health disorder diagnosis or who are receiving acute care for mental health disorder are guaranteed the same civil rights as any other citizen.
- Clients also have various specific rights, including the following.
  ○ Informed consent and the right to refuse treatment
  ○ Confidentiality
  ○ A written plan of care/treatment that includes discharge follow-up, as well as participation in the care plan and review of that plan
  ○ Communication with people outside the mental health facility, including family members, attorneys, and other health care professionals
  ○ Provision of adequate interpretive services if needed
  ○ Care provided with respect, dignity, and without discrimination
  ○ Freedom from harm related to physical or pharmacological restraint, seclusion, and any physical or mental abuse or neglect
  ○ A psychiatric advance directive that includes the client's treatment preferences in the event that an involuntary admission is necessary
  ○ Provision of care with the least restrictive interventions necessary to meet the client's needs without allowing them to be a threat to themselves or others

- Some legal issues regarding health care are decided in court using a specialized civil category called a tort. A tort is a wrongful act or injury committed by an entity or person against another person or another person's property. Torts can be used to decide liability issues, as well as intentional issues that can involve criminal penalties (abuse of a client).
- State laws can vary greatly. The nurse is responsible for knowing specific laws regarding client care within the state or states in which the nurse practices.
- The Mental Health Parity and Addiction Equity Act of 2008 requires insurance coverage for mental illness. The parity act, or state of equality, requires that coverage for mental health treatment must be considered and reviewed as any other medical treatment.

ETHICAL ISSUES FOR CLIENTS IN THE MENTAL HEALTH SETTING

- In comparison to laws, statutes, and regulations (enacted by local, state, or federal government), ethical issues are philosophical ideas regarding right and wrong.
- Nurses are frequently confronted with ethical dilemmas regarding client care (bioethical issues).
- The nurse can also experience situations where there will be a conflict between two or more courses of action, known as an ethical dilemma. The nurse should respond to these situations using the bioethical principles.
- Pharmacogenetic testing may be used to help predict side effects and efficacy with psychotropic medications, however, the FDA does not support genetic testing due to a lack of clinical evidence and research.
- Because ethics are philosophical and involve values and morals, there is frequently no clear-cut, simple resolution to an ethical dilemma.
- The nurse must use ethical principles to decide ethical issues. These include the following.

Beneficence: The quality of doing good; can be described as charity

> Example: A nurse helps a newly admitted client who has a psychotic disorder to feel safe in the environment of the mental health facility.

Autonomy: The client's right to make their own decisions. However, the client must accept the consequences of those decisions. The client must also respect the decisions of others.

> Example: Rather than giving advice to a client who has difficulty making decisions, a nurse helps the client explore all alternatives and arrive at a choice.

Justice: Fair and equal treatment for all

> Example: During a treatment team meeting, a nurse leads a discussion regarding whether or not two clients who broke the same facility rule were treated equally.

Fidelity: Loyalty and faithfulness to the client and to one's duty

> Example: A client asks a nurse to be present when they talk to their guardian for the first time in a year. The nurse remains with the client during this interaction.

Veracity: Honesty when dealing with a client

> Example: A client states, "You and that other staff member were talking about me, weren't you?" The nurse truthfully replies, "We were discussing ways to help you relate to the other clients in a more positive way."

CONFIDENTIALITY

- The client's right to privacy is protected by the Health Insurance Portability and Accountability Act (HIPAA) Privacy Rule of 2003.
- It is important to gain an understanding of the federal law and of state laws as they relate to confidentiality in specific health care facilities.
- The nurse should share information about the client, either verbal or written, only with those who are responsible for implementing the client's treatment plan. The nurse should not discuss client information in public places, and social media should never be used to discuss clients or their information.
- Only if the client provides consent should the nurse share information with other persons not involved in the client treatment plan.
- In most states, the Dead Man's Statute protects confidential information about individuals when they are not alive to speak for themselves.
- Specific mental health issues where health care professionals can break confidentiality include the duty to warn and protect third parties, and the reporting of child and vulnerable adult abuse.
- If the nurse becomes aware that a client's right to privacy is being violated, for example if a conversation in the elevator is overheard, they should immediately take action to stop the violation.

RESOURCES FOR SOLVING ETHICAL CLIENT ISSUES

- Code of Ethics for Nurses, found at the American Nurses Association's website.
- Patient Care Partnership, found at the American Hospital Association's website.
- The nurse practice act of a specific state
- Legal advice from attorneys
- Facility policies
- Other members of the health care team, including facility bioethics committee (if available)
- Members of the clergy and other spiritual or ethical counselors

TYPES OF ADMISSION TO A MENTAL HEALTH FACILITY

Informal admission: This is the least restrictive form of admission for treatment. The client does not pose a substantial threat to self or others. The client is free to leave the hospital at any time, even against medical advice.

Voluntary admission: The client or client's guardian chooses admission to a mental health facility in order to obtain treatment. This client is considered competent and so has the right to refuse medication and treatment. Before release, a client can be evaluated, and if deemed necessary, the care provider can initiate an involuntary admission.

Temporary emergency admission: The client is admitted for emergent mental health care due to the inability to make decisions regarding care. The medical health care provider can initiate the admission which is then evaluated by a mental health care provider. There must be a court hearing within 72 hr and another hearing in 7 to 21 hr depending up the state requirements.

Involuntary admission: The client enters the mental health facility against their will for an indefinite period of time. The admission is based on the client's need for psychiatric treatment, the risk of harm to self or others, or the inability to provide self-care. Qs

- The criteria for an involuntary admission include the following.
  - Manifestations of mental illness
  - Poses a danger to self or others
  - Demonstrates severe disability or inability to meet basic necessities including food, clothing, and shelter
  - Requires treatment but unable to seek it voluntarily related to the impact of the mental illness
- The number of physicians required to certify that the client's condition requires commitment varies from state to state (usually two). This can be imposed by a family member, legal guardian, primary care provider, or a mental health provider.
- The client can request a legal review of the admission at any time.
- For an involuntary admission, a psychiatric and legal review of the admission is required.
- Clients admitted under involuntary commitment are still considered competent and have the right to refuse treatment, including medication. The client who has been judged incompetent has a temporary or permanent guardian, usually a family member if possible, appointed by the court. The guardian can sign informed consent for the client. The guardian is expected to consider what the client would want if they were still competent.

CLIENT RIGHTS REGARDING SECLUSION AND RESTRAINT

- Nurses must know and follow federal/state/facility policies that govern the use of restraints.
- Use of seclusion rooms and/or restraints can be warranted and authorized for clients in some cases.
- Restraints are either physical or chemical (neuroleptic medication to calm the client).
- A client can voluntarily request a temporary timeout in cases in which the environment is disturbing or seems too stimulating. A timeout is different from prescribed seclusion because a timeout is by the request of the client.
- In general, the provider should prescribe seclusion and/or restraint for the shortest duration necessary, and only if less restrictive measures are not sufficient. They are for the physical protection of the client and/or the protection of other clients and staff. Qs
- Less restrictive measures
  - Verbal interventions (encouraging the client to calm down, asking the client for cooperation, active listening)
  - Diversion or redirection
  - Providing a calm, quiet environment
  - Offering a PRN medication (though technically a chemical restraint, medications are considered less restrictive than a mechanical restraint)
- The nurse should never use seclusion or restraint for the following.
  - Convenience of the staff
  - Punishment of the client
  - Clients who are extremely physically or mentally unstable
  - Clients who cannot tolerate the decreased stimulation of a seclusion room
- When the nurse has tried all other less restrictive means to prevent a client from harming self or others, the following must occur in order to use seclusion or restraint.
  - The provider must prescribe the seclusion or restraint in writing.
  - Time limits for seclusion or restraints are based upon the age of the client.
    - Age 18 years and older: 4 hr
    - Age 9 to 17 years: 2 hr
    - Age 8 years and younger: 1 hr
  - If the need for seclusion or restraint continues the provider must reassess the client and rewrite the prescription, specifying the type of restraint, every 24 hr or the frequency of time specified by facility policy.
  - Clients should never be secluded or left alone in a locked room, unsupervised or left in a prone or supine position. Continuous in-person or remote supervision is necessary.

- The facility protocol should identify the nursing responsibilities, including how often the client should be: Qᴇʙᴘ
  - Monitored (including for safety and physical needs), and the client's behavior documented
  - Offered food and fluid
  - Toileted
  - Monitored for cardiac, respiratory, and skin integrity, including vital signs
  - Monitored for pain
  - Complete documentation every 15 to 30 min (or according to facility policy) includes a description of the following.
    - Precipitating events and behavior of the client prior to seclusion or restraint
    - Alternative actions taken to avoid seclusion or restraint
    - The time treatment began
    - The client's current behavior, what foods or fluids were offered and taken, needs provided for, and vital signs
    - Medication administration
    - Time released from restraints
- The nurse can use seclusion or restraints without first obtaining a provider's written prescription if it is an emergency situation. If this emergency treatment is initiated, the nurse must obtain the written prescription within a specified period of time (usually 15 to 30 min).
- Restraint or seclusion must be discontinued when the client is exhibiting behavior that is safer and quieter. Once restraints or seclusion are discontinued, the nurse must obtain a new prescription before initiating restraints again.

TORT LAW IN THE MENTAL HEALTH SETTING

A tort is referred to as a civil wrong doing, in which monetary damages can potentially be awarded to the plaintiff (injured party) and collected from the defendant (responsible party).

INTENTIONAL TORTS

Intentional torts are willful actions that damage a client's property or violate client rights. Although intentional torts can occur in any health care setting, they are particularly likely to occur in mental health settings due to the increased likelihood of violence and client behavior that can be challenging to facility staff.

False imprisonment: Confining a client to a specific area (a seclusion room) physically, verbally, or using a chemical restraint when it is not part of the clients treatment (i.e., to prevent client harm to self or others) is considered false imprisonment.

Assault: Making a threat to a client's person (approaching the client in a threatening manner with a syringe in hand) is considered assault.

Battery: Touching a client in a harmful or offensive way is considered battery. This would occur if the nurse threatening the client with a syringe actually grabbed the client and gave an injection against the client's will.

Invasion of Privacy: Breaking confidences or by taking photographs without permission of the client.

UNINTENTIONAL TORTS

Unintentional torts are actions or inactions that cause unintended harm as a result of failing to meet one's duty of care in either a personal or professional situation.

Negligence: Failing to provide adequate care in a personal or professional situation when one has an obligation to do so. To be liable for negligence, it must be proven that the professional had a duty to protect, breached the duty, that the action or failure to act caused injury (proximate cause) and that the injury would not have happened anyway (cause in fact), and that damages occurred.

Malpractice: A type of professional negligence consisting of five elements:
- Breach of duty: Not meeting the standards of care
- Cause in fact and Proximate cause: "Did injury occur as a result of action taken by the nurses, or lack of action? Did the nurse foresee injury as a cause of their action or inaction?"
- Damages: Loss of earnings, property, or causing pain and suffering
- Duty: Understanding that specific knowledge and skills are needed for specialty nursing, like psychiatry.

DOCUMENTATION

It is vital to clearly and objectively document information related to violent or other unusual episodes. The nurse should document the following. Qᵒⁱ

Client behavior in a clear and objective manner

> Example: The client suddenly began to run down the hall with both hands in the air, screaming obscenities.

Staff response to disruptive, violent, or potentially harmful behavior (suicide threats or potential or actual harm to others), including timelines and the extent of response

> Example: The client states, "I'm going to pound (other client) into the ground." Client has picked up a chair and is standing 3 ft from other client with chair held over their head in both hands. Nurse calls for help. Client is immediately told by nurse, "Put down the chair, and back away from (the other person)." Other client moved away to safe area. Five other staff members respond to verbal call for help within 30 seconds and stood several yards from client. Client then put the chair down, quietly turned around, walked to their room, and sat on the bed.

Time the nurse notified the provider and any prescriptions received.

Application Exercises

1. A nurse hears a newly licensed nurse discussing a client's hallucinations in the hallway with another nurse. Which of the following actions should the nurse take first?
   A. Notify the nurse manager.
   B. Tell the nurse to stop discussing the behavior.
   C. Provide an in-service program about confidentiality.
   D. Complete an incident report.

2. A nurse in an emergency mental health facility is caring for a group of clients. The nurse should identify that which of the following clients requires a temporary emergency admission?
   A. A client who has schizophrenia with delusions of grandeur.
   B. A client who has manifestations of depression and attempted suicide a year ago.
   C. A client who has borderline personality disorder and assaulted a homeless man with a metal rod.
   D. A client who has bipolar disorder and paces quickly around the room while talking to themselves.

3. A nurse is caring for a client who is in mechanical restraints. Which of the following statements should the nurse include in the documentation? (Select all that apply.)
   A. "Client ate most of their breakfast."
   B. "Client was offered 8 oz of water every hr."
   C. "Client shouted obscenities at assistive personnel."
   D. "Client received chlorpromazine 15 mg by mouth at 1000."
   E. "Client acted out after lunch."

4. A nurse decides to put a client who has a psychotic disorder in seclusion overnight because the unit is very short-staffed, and the client frequently fights with other clients. The nurse's actions are an example of which of the following torts?
   A. Invasion of privacy
   B. False imprisonment
   C. Assault
   D. Battery

Active Learning Scenario

A nurse in a mental health facility is caring for an adult client who has bipolar disorder. The client becomes violent and begins throwing objects at other clients. After calling for assistance, what actions should the nurse take next? Use the ATI Active Learning Template: Basic Concept to complete this item.

NURSING INTERVENTIONS: Describe at least four actions the nurse can take to manage the client's behavior before applying mechanical restraints. Include rationales for the actions.

1. B. **CORRECT:** The greatest risk to this client is an invasion of privacy through the sharing of confidential information in a public place. The first action to take is to tell the newly licensed nurse to stop discussing the client's hallucinations in a public location. Notify the nurse manager if the client's right to privacy is violated. However, there is another action to take first. Provide an in-service program for staff about confidentiality. However, there is another action to take first. Complete an incident report about the violation of the client's right to privacy. However, there is another action to take first.

   Ⓝ *NCLEX® Connection: Coordinated Care, Confidentiality/ Information Security*

2. C. **CORRECT:** When analyzing cues, the nurse should identify a client who is a current danger to self or others is a candidate for a temporary emergency admission. The presence of delusions does not constitute a clear reason for a temporary emergency admission unless they present a danger for the client or others. Clinical findings of depression do not constitute a clear reason for a temporary emergency admission unless the client is currently at risk for suicide. The presence of pacing does not constitute a clear reason for a temporary emergency admission.

   Ⓝ *NCLEX® Connection: Psychosocial Integrity, Crisis Intervention*

3. B, C, D. **CORRECT:** The nurse should include the following statements in the documentation for a client who has mechanical restraints: The amount and frequency of fluids offered is objective data that should be documented when caring for a client in mechanical restraints. A description of the client's verbal communication is objective data that should be documented when caring for a client in mechanical restraints. The dosage and time of medication administration is objective data that should be documented when caring for a client in mechanical restraints.

   Ⓝ *NCLEX® Connection: Safety and Infection Control, Least Restrictive Restraints and Safety Devices*

4. B. **CORRECT:** When taking actions, the nurse should recognize a civil wrong that violates a client's civil rights is a tort. In this case, it is false imprisonment, which is the confining of a client to a specific area (a seclusion room) if the reason for such confinement is for the convenience of staff. Invasion of privacy is the sharing or obtaining of the client's confidential information without the client's consent. Assault is making a threat to the client's person. Battery involves causing intentional, physical harm to clients.

   Ⓝ *NCLEX® Connection: Safety and Infection Control, Least Restrictive Restraints and Safety Devices*

Using the ATI Active Learning Template: Basic Concept

NURSING INTERVENTIONS

- Tell the client calmly to sit down. Verbal intervention is the least restrictive method when dealing with an aggressive client.
- Provide the client with a decreased-stimulation environment and attempt diversion or redirection. These interventions are less restrictive than seclusion or restraint and the nurse should attempt these interventions prior to more restrictive actions.
- Offer the client a PRN medication (diazepam). It can be necessary for the nurse to administer diazepam to calm the client and is considered less restrictive than mechanical restraints.
- Place the client in a monitored seclusion room. It can become necessary to place the client in seclusion if the client persists in the behavior after attempting less restrictive interventions.
- If other interventions are unsuccessful, obtain a prescription for mechanical restraints. Follow facility policy for the application of restraints and the monitoring and documentation required for the client's care.

Ⓝ *NCLEX® Connection: Psychosocial Integrity, Behavioral Management*

UNIT 1   FOUNDATIONS FOR MENTAL HEALTH NURSING

CHAPTER 3 *Effective Communication*

Communication is a complex process of sending, receiving, and comprehending messages between two or more people. It is a dynamic and ongoing process that creates a unique experience between the participants.

Communicating effectively is a skill that the nurse develops. Nurses use communication when providing care to establish relationships, demonstrate caring, obtain information, and assist with changing behaviors. Foundational to the nurse-client relationship is therapeutic communication.

BASIC COMMUNICATION

BASIC LEVELS OF COMMUNICATION Qpcc

Intrapersonal communication: Communication that occurs within an individual. Also identified as "self-talk." This occurs within one's self and is the internal discussion that takes place when an individual is thinking thoughts and not outwardly verbalizing them. In nursing, intrapersonal communication allows nurses to perform a self-assessment of their values or beliefs prior to caring for a client whose diagnosis can trigger an emotional response.

Interpersonal communication: Communication that occurs one-on-one with another individual. In nursing, interpersonal communication is used when the nurse obtains a psychosocial history from a client or when listening to a client discuss their feelings.

Small-group communication: Communication that occurs between two or more people in a small group. In nursing, small-group communication allows the nurse to discuss a change in the client's behavior with the health care team or discuss concerns with clients during a group therapy session.

Public communication: Communication that occurs within large groups of people. In nursing, this commonly occurs during educational endeavors where the nurse is collaborating with the RN to educate a large group of individuals. For example, the nurse can reinforce about suicide prevention with high school students at a school assembly.

Electronic communication: Using technology for secure messaging and timely communication between client and health care provider. This type of communication helps clients stay engaged in their care and develop ongoing relationships with health care providers.

Verbal communication

Vocabulary
- These are the words that are used to communicate either a written or a spoken message.
- Limited vocabulary or speaking a language other than English can make it difficult for the nurse to communicate with the client. Use of medical jargon can decrease client understanding.

Denotative/connotative meaning
- When communicating, participants must share meanings.
- Words that have multiple meanings can cause miscommunication if they are interpreted differently.

Clarity/brevity
- The shortest, simplest communication is usually most effective.
- The client can have difficulty understanding communication that is long and complex.

Timing/relevance
- Knowing when to communicate allows the receiver to be more attentive to the message.
- Communicating with a client who is in pain or distracted will make it difficult for the nurse to convey the message.

Pacing
- The rate of speech can communicate a meaning to the receiver.
- Speaking rapidly can communicate the impression that the nurse is in a rush and does not have time for the client.

Intonation
- The tone of voice can communicate a variety of feelings.
- The nurse can communicate feelings (acceptance, judgment, and dislike) through tone of voice.

Nonverbal communication

Nurses should be aware of how they communicate nonverbally. The nurse should monitor the client's nonverbal communications for the meaning being conveyed, remembering that culture impacts interpretation. Nonverbal communication can have more impact on the message compared to the verbal words.

It is important for the nurse to consider how emotions like anger, depression, and anxiety may can express as an incongruency for the client experiencing a mental illness. The nurse should re-assess mood and clarify if they are unsure how a client is feeling.

Attention to the following behaviors is important, as it is compared to the verbal message being conveyed.
- Appearance
- Posture
- Gait
- Facial expressions
- Eye contact
- Gestures
- Sounds
- Territoriality
- Personal space
- Silence

The nurse should use verbal techniques to clarify client emotions and monitor client behavior for the following nonverbal cues.

- **Affect**: Frowning; lack of expression; grimacing; pursed lips; raised or lowered eyebrows; biting, licking, smacking lips; nose scrunching
- **Appearance**: Sudden disrobing; clothing that is incongruent to current temperature; disheveled grooming
- **Autonomic Response**: Visible brow or palm perspiration; pupil dilation; facial flushing or paleness; increased respirations
- **Body Behaviors**: Gait; posture; hand clenching; rocking; psychomotor agitation
- **Eye Movement**: Suspicious; squinting; open with minimal blinking

THERAPEUTIC COMMUNICATION

Therapeutic communication is the purposeful use of communication to build and maintain helping relationships with clients, families, and significant others. Therapeutic communication is essential when caring for a client who has a mental health disorder because of the emotional as well as the physical effects of the disorder on the client. Qpcc

- The nurse uses interactive, purposeful communication skills to
  - Elicit and attend to the client's thoughts, feelings, concerns, and needs.
  - Express empathy and genuine concern for the client's and family's issues.
  - Obtain information and give feedback about the client's condition.
  - Intervene to promote functional behavior and effective interpersonal relationships.
  - Monitor the client's progress toward goals and outcomes.
- Children and older adults frequently require adapted techniques to enhance communication. Ⓖ
- Effective use of the nursing process depends on therapeutic communication between the nurse, the client, the client's family, and the interprofessional team.

CHARACTERISTICS

- Client centered: not social or reciprocal
- Purposeful, planned, and goal-directed

ESSENTIAL COMPONENTS

Time
- Plan for and allow adequate time to communicate.
- Clients who have certain mental health disorders (major depressive disorder or schizophrenia) can require a longer period of time to respond to questions.

Attending behaviors or active listening
- These are nonverbal means of conveying interest in another.
- Eye contact typically conveys interest and respect but varies by situation and culture.
- Body language and posture can demonstrate level of comfort and ease.
- Vocal quality enhances rapport and emphasizes particular topics or issues.
- Verbal tracking provides feedback by restating or summarizing a client's statements.

Caring attitude: Show concern and facilitate an emotional connection with the client and the client's family.

Honesty: Be open, direct, truthful, and sincere.

Trust: Demonstrate reliability without doubt or question.

Empathy: Convey an objective awareness and understanding of the feelings, emotions, and behaviors of others, including trying to envision what it must be like to be in the position of the client and the client's family.

Nonjudgmental attitude: This is a display of acceptance that will encourage open, honest communication.

NURSING PROCESS

DATA COLLECTION

- Collect data about verbal and nonverbal communication needs.
- Identify any cultural considerations that can impact communication (the use of eye contact or perception of personal space or touch). Qpcc
- Recognize congruency between the verbal and nonverbal message.
- Consider the client's developmental level and how communication should be adapted.

CHILDREN
- Use simple, straightforward language.
- Be aware of own nonverbal messages, as children are sensitive to nonverbal communication.
- Enhance communication by being at the child's eye level.
- Incorporate play in interactions.
- Be aware of the child's level of development. Responses may be concrete until abstract thinking is developed.

ADOLESCENTS
- Determine how the adolescent perceives the mental health diagnosis. Is the adolescent at risk for refusal of treatment due to a desire to be "normal"?
- Identify if the mental health diagnosis affects the client's relationship with their peers or their ability to explore their identity.

OLDER ADULT CLIENTS Ⓖ
- Recognize that the client might require amplification.
- Minimize distractions, and face the client when speaking.
- Allow plenty of time for the client to respond.
- When impaired communication is present, ask for input from caregivers or family to determine the extent of the deficits and how best to communicate.

PLANNING

- Minimize distractions.
- Provide for privacy.
- Identify mutually agreed-upon client outcomes.
- Set priorities according to the client's needs.
- Plan for adequate time for interventions.

IMPLEMENTATION

- Explain the purpose of writing notes or recording notes into an electronic health record at the beginning of the interview.
- Establish a trusting nurse-client relationship. The client feels more at ease during the implementation phase once a helping relationship is established.
  - Reiterate the client's right to privacy and confidentiality. Explain exceptions to confidentiality.
  - **Diversity, equity, and inclusion (DEI)** are essential qualities that a nurse considers when building rapport in the professional nurse-client relationship.
- Provide empathetic responses and explanations to the client by using observations and providing hope, humor, and information.
- Manipulate the environment to decrease distractions.
- If in a private area, ensure accessibility to help in case of an emergency.
- Bias-free language.
  - Focus on relevant characteristics
  - Acknowledge relevant differences that do exist
  - Acknowledge people's humanity ("What pronouns do you prefer?")
  - Avoid false hierarchies (Careful use of the word "normal.")

EFFECTIVE COMMUNICATION SKILLS AND TECHNIQUES

Silence: Silence allows time for meaningful reflection.

Active listening: The nurse is able to hear, observe, and understand what the client communicates and to provide feedback.

Questions: Questions allow the nurse to obtain specific or additional information from the client.
- **Open-ended questions**: Facilitates spontaneous responses and interactive discussion
- **Closed-ended questions:** Helpful if used sparingly during the initial interaction to obtain specific data. Avoid using repeated closed-ended questions which can block further communication.
- **Projective questions:** Uses "what if" or similar questions to assist clients in exploring feelings and to gain greater understanding of problems and possible solutions
- **Presupposition questions**: Explores the client's life goals or motivations by presenting a hypothetical situation in which the client no longer has the mental health disorder

Clarifying techniques: This technique is used to determine if the message received was accurate.
- **Restating** uses the client's exact words.
- **Reflecting** directs the focus back to the client in order for the client to examine his feelings.
- **Paraphrasing** restates the client's feelings and thoughts for the client to confirm what has been communicated.
- **Exploring** allows the nurse to gather more information regarding important topics mentioned by the client.

Offering general leads, broad opening statements: This encourages the client to determine where the communication can start and to continue talking.

Showing acceptance and recognition: This technique acknowledges the nurse's interest and nonjudgmental attitude.

Focusing: This technique helps the client to concentrate on what is important.

Giving information: This technique provides details that the client might need for decision making.

Presenting reality: This technique is used to help the client focus on what is actually happening and to dispel delusions, hallucinations, or faulty beliefs.

Summarizing: Summarizing emphasizes important points and reviews what has been discussed.

Offering self: Use of this technique demonstrates a willingness to spend time with the client. Indicates to the client that the nurse has genuine concern.

Touch: If appropriate, therapeutic touch communicates caring and can provide comfort to the client.

Seating: A client experiencing manifestations of hyperactivity, or increased anxiety, may have difficulties in communicating while sitting. Consider walking around the room or unit to improve communication adherence.

Motivational interviewing: A style of communication that assists clients in developing motivation to resolve insecurities and ambivalent feelings towards behavior change.

BARRIERS TO EFFECTIVE COMMUNICATION

- Asking irrelevant personal questions
- Offering personal opinions
- Giving advice
- Giving false reassurance
- Minimizing feelings
- Changing the topic
- Asking "why" questions
- Offering value judgments
- Excessive questioning
- Rapid questioning
- Giving approval or disapproval

Application Exercises

1. A charge nurse is conducting a class on therapeutic communication with a group of newly licensed nurses. Which of the following aspects of communication should the nurse identify as a component of verbal communication?

    A. Personal space

    B. Posture

    C. Eye contact

    D. Intonation

2. A nurse in a mental health practitioner's office is communicating with a client. The client states, "I can't sleep. I stay up all night." The nurse responds, "You are having difficulty sleeping?" Which of the following therapeutic communication techniques is the nurse demonstrating?

    A. Offering general leads

    B. Summarizing

    C. Focusing

    D. Restating

3. A nurse is talking with the caregiver of a child who has demonstrated recent changes in behavior and mood. When the caregiver of the child asks the nurse for reassurance about their child's condition, which of the following responses should the nurse make?

    A. "I think your child is getting better. What have you noticed?"

    B. "I'm sure everything will be okay. It just takes time to heal."

    C. "I'm not sure what's wrong. Have you asked the doctor about your concerns?"

    D. "I understand you're concerned. Let's discuss what concerns you specifically."

4. A nurse is communicating with a client who was admitted for treatment of a substance use disorder. Which of the following communication techniques should the nurse identify as a barrier to therapeutic communication?

    A. Offering advice

    B. Reflecting

    C. Listening attentively

    D. Giving information

Active Learning Scenario

A nurse in a mental health facility is preparing to conduct a class with older adult clients on grief and loss. Use the ATI Active Learning Template: Basic Concept to complete this item.

NURSING INTERVENTIONS: Describe at least four verbal or nonverbal communication interventions the nurse should employ when working with older adult clients.

Application Exercises Key

1. D. **CORRECT:** When recognizing cues, the nurse should identify that intonation is a component of verbal communication. Personal space, posture, and eye contact are components of nonverbal communication.

    Ⓝ *NCLEX® Connection: Psychosocial Integrity, Therapeutic Communication*

2. D. **CORRECT:** The nurse is using the therapeutic communication technique of restating which allows the nurse to repeat the main idea expressed by the client. Offering general leads lets the nurse to take the direction of the discussion. Summarizing enables the nurse to bring together important points of discussion to enhance understanding. Focusing concentrates the attention on one single point.

    Ⓝ *NCLEX® Connection: Psychosocial Integrity, Therapeutic Communication*

3. A. This nontherapeutic response interjects the nurse's opinion and can cause the caregiver to withhold their thoughts and feelings.

    B. This nontherapeutic response interjects the nurse's opinion and provides false reassurance which can cause the caregiver to withhold their thoughts and feelings.

    C. This nontherapeutic response avoids addressing the caregiver's concerns directly and indicates disinterest by the nurse for wanting to discuss the concerns with the parents.

    D. **CORRECT:** This therapeutic response reflects upon, and accepts, the caregivers' feelings, and it allows them to clarify what they are feeling.

    Ⓝ *NCLEX® Connection: Psychosocial Integrity, Therapeutic Communication*

4. A. **CORRECT:** Offering advice to a client is a barrier to therapeutic communication that should be avoided. Advice tends to interfere with the client's ability to make personal decisions and choices. The technique of reflection directs the focus back to the client in order for the client to examine his feelings. The skill of active listening is an important therapeutic technique to help hear and understand the information and messages the client is trying to convey. Giving information informs the client of needed information to assist in the treatment planning process.

    Ⓝ *NCLEX® Connection: Psychosocial Integrity, Therapeutic Communication*

Active Learning Scenario Key

Using the ATI Active Learning Template: Basic Concept

NURSING INTERVENTIONS
- Recognize that the client might require amplification.
- Minimize distractions, and face the client when speaking.
- Allow plenty of time for the client to respond.
- When impaired communication is present, ask for input from caregivers or family to determine the extent of the deficits and how best to communicate.
- Provide for privacy.

Ⓝ *NCLEX® Connection: Psychosocial Integrity, Therapeutic Communication*

UNIT 1   FOUNDATIONS FOR MENTAL HEALTH NURSING

CHAPTER 4
Stress and Defense Mechanisms

Stress can result from a change in one's environment that is threatening, causes challenges, or is perceived as damaging to that person's well-being. Stress causes anxiety. Dysfunctional behavior can occur when a defense mechanism is used as a response to anxiety.

Individuals can use defense mechanisms as a way to manage conflict in response to anxiety. Defense mechanisms are reversible, and the client can use them in either an adaptive or maladaptive manner. Adaptive use of defense mechanisms helps people to achieve their goals in acceptable ways and reduce anxiety. Defense mechanisms become maladaptive when they interfere with functioning, relationships, and orientation to reality and are used in excess. It is important that the defense mechanism used is appropriate to the situation, and that an individual uses a variety of defense mechanisms, rather than having the same reaction to every stressful situation.

Defense mechanisms

Altruism and sublimation are defense mechanisms that are always healthy. Other defense mechanisms can be used in a healthy manner. However, they can become maladaptive if used inappropriately or repetitively. Consider the frequency, intensity, and duration of use of the client's defense mechanisms to determine whether they are adaptive or maladaptive.

When a client is defensive or exhibiting defense mechanisms, the goal is to maintain a therapeutic relationship that is based on trust, focuses on well-being with healthy boundaries, and assists the client toward a healthy coping strategy.

Altruism

Dealing with anxiety by reaching out to others

ADAPTIVE USE: A nurse who lost a family member in a fire is a volunteer firefighter.

MALADAPTIVE USE: n/a

Sublimation

Dealing with unacceptable feelings or impulses by unconsciously substituting acceptable forms of expression

ADAPTIVE USE: A person who has feelings of anger and hostility toward their work supervisor sublimates those feelings by working out vigorously at the gym during their lunch period.

MALADAPTIVE USE: n/a

Suppression

Voluntarily denying unpleasant thoughts and feelings

ADAPTIVE USE: A student puts off thinking about a fight they had with a friend so they can focus on a test.

MALADAPTIVE USE: A person who has lost their job states they will worry about paying bills next week.

Repression

Unconsciously putting unacceptable ideas, thoughts, and emotions out of awareness

ADAPTIVE USE: A person preparing to give a speech unconsciously forgets about the time when they were young and kids laughed at them while on stage.

MALADAPTIVE USE: A person who has a fear of the dentist continually forgets to go to their dental appointments.

Regression

Sudden use of childlike or primitive behaviors that do not correlate with the person's current developmental level

ADAPTIVE USE: A young child temporarily wets the bed when they learn that their pet died.

MALADAPTIVE USE: A person who has a disagreement with a co-worker begins throwing things at their office.

Displacement

Shifting feelings related to an object, person, or situation to another less threatening object, person, or situation

ADAPTIVE USE: An adolescent angrily punches a punching bag after losing a game.

MALADAPTIVE USE: A person who is angry about losing their job destroys their child's favorite toy.

Reaction formation

Overcompensating or demonstrating the opposite behavior of what is felt

ADAPTIVE USE: A person who is trying to quit smoking repeatedly talks to adolescents about the dangers of nicotine.

MALADAPTIVE USE: A person who dislikes their neighbor tells others what a great neighbor she is.

Undoing

Performing an act to make up for prior behavior (most commonly seen in children)

ADAPTIVE USE: An adolescent completes their chores without being prompted after having an argument with their parent.

MALADAPTIVE USE: An individual buys their significant other flowers and gifts after an incident of partner abuse.

Rationalization

Creating reasonable and acceptable explanations for unacceptable behavior

ADAPTIVE USE: An adolescent says, "They must already have a boyfriend" when rejected by another adolescent.

MALADAPTIVE USE: A young adult explains they had to drive themselves home from a party after drinking alcohol because they had to feed the dog.

Dissociation

Creating a temporary compartmentalization or lack of connection between the person's identity, memory, or how they perceive the environment

ADAPTIVE USE: A parent blocks out the distracting noise from their children in order to focus while driving in traffic.

MALADAPTIVE USE: A person forgets their identity after a sexual assault.

Denial

Pretending the truth is not reality to manage unpleasant, anxiety-causing thoughts or feelings

ADAPTIVE USE: A person initially says, "No, that can't be true" when told they have cancer.

MALADAPTIVE USE: A parent who is informed that their child was killed in combat tells everyone one month later that the child is coming home for the holidays.

Compensation

Emphasizing strengths to make up for weaknesses

ADAPTIVE USE: An adolescent who is physically unable to play contact sports excels in academic competitions.

MALADAPTIVE USE: A person who is shy learns computer skills to avoid socialization.

Identification

Conscious or unconscious assumption of the characteristics of another individual or group

ADAPTIVE USE: A child who has a chronic illness pretends to be a nurse for their dolls.

MALADAPTIVE USE: A child who observes their parent be abusive toward the other parent becomes a bully at school.

Intellectualization

Separation of emotions and logical facts when analyzing or coping with a situation or event

ADAPTIVE USE: A law enforcement officer blocks out the emotional aspect of a crime so they can objectively focus on the investigation.

MALADAPTIVE USE: A person who learns they have a terminal illness focuses on creating a will and financial matters rather than acknowledging their grief.

Conversion

Responding to stress through the unconscious development of physical manifestations not caused by a physical illness

ADAPTIVE USE: n/a

MALADAPTIVE USE: A person experiences deafness after their partner tells them they want a divorce.

Splitting

Demonstrating an inability to reconcile negative and positive attributes of self or others

ADAPTIVE USE: n/a

MALADAPTIVE USE: A client tells a nurse that she is the only one who cares about her, yet the following day, the same client refuses to talk to the nurse.

Projection

Attributing one's unacceptable thoughts and feelings onto another who does not have them

ADAPTIVE USE: n/a

MALADAPTIVE USE: A married client who is attracted to another person accuses their partner of having an extramarital affair.

Anxiety

Anxiety is viewed on a continuum with increasing levels of anxiety leading to decreasing ability to function.

Normal

A healthy life force that is necessary for survival, normal anxiety motivates people to take action.

> For example, a potentially violent situation occurs on the mental health unit, and the nurse moves rapidly to defuse the situation. The anxiety experienced by the nurse during the situation helped them perform quickly and efficiently.

Acute (immediate state)

This level of anxiety is precipitated by an imminent loss or change that threatens one's sense of security.

> For example, the sudden death of a loved one precipitates an acute state of anxiety.

Chronic (sustained trait)

This level of anxiety is one that usually develops over time, often starting in childhood. The adult who experiences chronic anxiety might display that anxiety in physical manifestations (fatigue, frequent headaches).

DATA COLLECTION

Identifying a client's level of anxiety is basic to therapeutic intervention in any setting.

TOXIC STRESS RESPONSE

Manifestations of biological and neurological changes that are a result of sustained toxic stress. A client may exhibit a variety of somatic symptoms such as gastrointestinal discomfort, body aches, and shortness of breath. Alterations in executive functioning, including language and problem solving, may also be present. The nurse should especially be aware of pediatric clients who may be exhibiting manifestations of toxic stress as this may be related to Adverse Childhood Experiences like neglect, exposure to violence, and family economic hardships.

LEVELS OF ANXIETY

Mild

- Mild anxiety occurs in the normal experience of everyday living.
- It increases one's ability to perceive reality.
- There is an identifiable cause of the anxiety.
- Other characteristics include a vague feeling of mild discomfort, restlessness, irritability, impatience, and apprehension.
- Client can demonstrate tapping of foot or finger, chewing their lip, or other restless behavior to help relieve tension.

Moderate

- Moderate anxiety occurs when mild anxiety escalates.
- Slightly reduced perception and processing of information occurs, and selective inattention can occur.
- Ability to think clearly is hampered, but learning and problem-solving can still occur.
- Other characteristics include concentration difficulties, tiredness, pacing, change in voice pitch, voice tremors, shakiness, and increased heart rate and respiratory rate.
- The client can report somatic manifestations including headaches, backache, urinary urgency and frequency, and insomnia.
- The client who has this type of anxiety usually benefits from the direction of others.

Severe

- Perceptual field is greatly reduced with distorted perceptions.
- Learning and problem-solving do not occur.
- Functioning is effective; behaviors are automatic.
- Other characteristics include confusion, feelings of impending doom, hyperventilation, tachycardia, withdrawal, loud and rapid speech, and aimless activity.
- The client who has severe anxiety usually is not able to take direction from others.

Panic

- Panic-level anxiety is characterized by markedly disturbed behavior.
- The client is not able to process what is occurring in the environment and can lose touch with reality.
- The client experiences extreme fright and horror.
- The client experiences severe hyperactivity, flight, or immobility.
- Other characteristics can include dysfunction in speech, dilated pupils, severe shakiness, severe withdrawal, inability to sleep, delusions, and hallucinations.

PATIENT-CENTERED CARE

Practices and therapies for the alleviation of stress and anxiety foster a mind-to-body and body-to-mind approach to manage manifestations by producing psychophysiological effects that reduce the effects of the stressor. Some effective stress reducing activities include aerobic exercise, moderating caffeine intake, listening to music, and improving the quality of sleep. Nursing interventions are implemented according to the level of anxiety that a client is experiencing.

NURSING INTERVENTIONS

Mild to moderate anxiety

Use active listening to demonstrate willingness to help, and use specific communication techniques (open-ended questions, giving broad openings, exploring, and seeking clarification).
THERAPEUTIC INTENT: Encourages the client to express feelings, develop trust, and identify the source of the anxiety.

Provide a calm presence, recognizing the client's distress.
THERAPEUTIC INTENT: Assists the client to focus and to begin to problem solve.

Evaluate past coping mechanisms.
THERAPEUTIC INTENT: Assists the client to identify adaptive and maladaptive coping mechanisms.

Explore alternatives to problem situations.
THERAPEUTIC INTENT: Offers options for problem-solving.

Encourage participation in activities, such as exercise, that can temporarily relieve feelings of inner tension.
THERAPEUTIC INTENT: Provides an outlet for pent-up tension, promotes endorphin release, and improves mental well-being.

Severe to panic anxiety

Provide an environment that meets the physical and safety needs of the client. Remain with the client and remain calm.
THERAPEUTIC INTENT: Minimizes risk to the client, who might be unaware of the need for basic things (fluids, food, sleep). Qs

Provide a quiet environment with minimal stimulation.
THERAPEUTIC INTENT: Helps to prevent intensification of the current level of anxiety.

Use medications, seclusion, or restraint, but only after less restrictive interventions have failed to decrease anxiety to safer levels.
THERAPEUTIC INTENT: Medications and/or restraint might be necessary to prevent harm to the client, other clients, and providers.

Encourage gross motor activities, such as walking and other forms of exercise.
THERAPEUTIC INTENT: Provides an outlet for pent-up tension, promotes endorphin release, and improves mental well-being.

Set limits by using firm, short, and simple statements. Repetition can be necessary. Speak slowly and in a low pitched voice.
THERAPEUTIC INTENT: Can minimize risk to the client and providers. Clear, simple communication facilitates understanding.

Direct the client to acknowledge reality and focus on what is present in the environment.
THERAPEUTIC INTENT: Focusing on reality assists with reducing the client's anxiety level.

Application Exercises

1. A nurse is caring for a client who smokes and has lung cancer. The client reports, "I'm coughing because I have that cold that everyone has been getting." The nurse should identify that the client is using which of the following defense mechanisms?
   A. Reaction formation
   B. Denial
   C. Displacement
   D. Sublimation

2. A nurse is reinforcing preoperative teaching with a client who was informed of the need for emergency surgery. The client has a respiratory rate 30/min, and says, "This is difficult to comprehend. I feel shaky and nervous." The nurse should identify that the client is experiencing which of the following levels of anxiety?
   A. Mild
   B. Moderate
   C. Severe
   D. Panic

3. A nurse is caring for a client who is experiencing moderate anxiety. Which of the following actions should the nurse take when trying to reinforce necessary information to the client? (Select all that apply.)
   A. Reassure the client that everything will be okay.
   B. Discuss prior use of coping mechanisms with the client.
   C. Ignore the client's anxiety so that she will not be embarrassed.
   D. Demonstrate a calm manner while using simple and clear directions.
   E. Gather information from the client using closed-ended questions.

Active Learning Scenario

A nurse is caring for a client who has severe anxiety. Use the ATI Active Learning Template: Basic Concept to complete this item.

NURSING INTERVENTIONS: Identify four nursing interventions that the nurse can use to assist the client who is experiencing severe anxiety.

Application Exercises Key

1. **CORRECT:** B

   When assessing the client, the nurse should identify this is an example of denial, which is pretending the truth is not reality to manage the anxiety of acknowledging what is real. This is not an example of reaction formation, which is overcompensating or demonstrating the opposite behavior of what is felt. This is not an example of displacement, which is shifting feelings related to an object, person, or situation to another less threatening object, person, or situation. This is not an example of sublimation, which is dealing with unacceptable feelings or impulses by unconsciously substituting acceptable forms of expression.

   Ⓝ *NCLEX® Connection: Psychosocial Integrity, Mental Health Concepts*

2. **CORRECT:** B

   When evaluation data, the nurse should identify that moderate anxiety decreases problem-solving and may hamper the client's ability to understand information. Vital signs may increase somewhat, and the client is visibly anxious. In mild anxiety, the client's ability to understand information may actually increase. Severe anxiety causes restlessness, decreased perception, and an inability to take direction. During a panic attack, the person is completely distracted, unable to function, and may lose touch with reality.

   Ⓝ *NCLEX® Connection: Psychosocial Integrity, Behavioral Management*

3. **CORRECT:** B, D

   When taking action, the nurse should discuss the prior use of coping mechanisms that assists the client in identifying ways of effectively coping with the current stressor. Providing a calm presence assists the client in feeling secure and promotes relaxation. Clients experiencing moderate levels of anxiety often benefit from the direction of others. Recognizing the client's current level of anxiety assists the client to begin the process of problem solving. Providing false reassurance is an example of nontherapeutic communication. Using open-ended questions for client communication encourages the client to express feelings and identify the source of the anxiety.

   Ⓝ *NCLEX® Connection: Psychosocial Integrity, Behavioral Management*

Active Learning Scenario Key

Using the ATI Active Learning Template: Basic Concept

NURSING INTERVENTIONS
- Provide an environment that meets the physical and safety needs of the client. Remain with the client.
- Provide a quiet environment with minimal stimulation.
- Use medications and restraint, but only after less restrictive interventions have failed to decrease anxiety to safer levels.
- Encourage gross motor activities, such as walking and other forms of exercise.
- Set limits by using firm, short, and simple statements. Repetition may be necessary.
- Direct the client to acknowledge reality and focus on what is present in the environment.

Ⓝ *NCLEX® Connection: Psychosocial Integrity, Behavioral Management*

UNIT 1   FOUNDATIONS FOR MENTAL HEALTH NURSING

CHAPTER 5 # Creating and Maintaining a Therapeutic and Safe Environment

Therapeutic encounters can occur in any setting if a nurse is sensitive to a client's needs and uses effective communication skills.

The therapeutic nurse-client relationship is foundational to nursing care in a mental health setting.

The therapeutic nurse-client relationship differs from other social and intimate relationships.

A therapeutic nurse-client relationship has the following characteristics.

- Purposeful and goal-directed
- Well-defined with clear boundaries
- Structured to meet the client's needs
- Culturally competent practice and care
- Characterized by an interpersonal process that is safe, confidential, reliable, and consistent

MILIEU THERAPY

Milieu therapy creates an environment that is supportive, therapeutic, and safe. Milieu therapy can also be referred to as a therapeutic community or therapeutic environment.

- Management of the milieu refers to the management of the total environment, physical and psychosocial, of the mental health unit in order to provide the least amount of stress, ensure client and staff safety, managing behavioral crisis, while promoting a client's belief in their own abilities toward recovery and improved functioning.
- The goal is that while the client is in this therapeutic environment, the client will learn the tools necessary to cope adaptively, interact more effectively and appropriately, and strengthen relationship skills. The hope is that the client will use these tools in all other aspects of their life.
- The nurse, as manager of care, is responsible for structuring and/or implementing aspects of the therapeutic milieu within the mental health facility.
- One structure of the therapeutic milieu is regular community meetings, which include both the clients and the nursing staff.

CHARACTERISTICS OF THE THERAPEUTIC MILIEU

Physical environment

Setting should be clean, safe, and orderly.
The setting should include comfortable furniture placed so that it promotes interaction, solitary spaces for reading and thinking alone, comfortable places conducive to meals, and quiet areas for sleeping.
Color scheme and overall design should be appropriate for the client's age.
Furniture, walls, floors, and decor should consist of materials that are considered safe, easy to clean, and attractive.
Consideration should be given to traffic-flow, as well as movement of clients and staff.
Adjust environment stimulation so appropriate for client condition such as noise level and appropriate lighting.
Fostering least restrictive environment based on client needs and situation.

Psychosocial environment

Clients should feel safe from harm (self-harm, as well as harm from the disruptive behaviors of other clients).
Clients should feel cared for and accepted by the health care team by providing a respectful, empathetic approach in all interpersonal interactions.
Clients should experience a therapeutic, healing climate for activities and therapies that focus on improved quality of life and recovery.

Health care team member responsibilities

Promote client care which is a balance in client autonomy and independence with their responsibility and ability for self-control, self-care and individual growth.
Treat clients as individuals, including
- Provide fair, equitable treatment for all clients.
- Allow choices for clients within the daily routine and within individual treatment plans.
- Model good social behavior for clients, such as respecting the rights of others.
- Work cooperatively as a team to provide care.
- Maintain boundaries with clients.
- Maintain a professional appearance and demeanor.
- Promote safe and satisfying peer interactions among the clients.
- Practice open communication techniques with health team members and clients.
- Promote feelings of self-worth and hope for the future.
- Ensure a safe and predictable environment in which a client can develop coping skills, problem-solving abilities, and relationship skills. Ideally, every aspect of a client's treatment environment

THERAPEUTIC NURSE-CLIENT RELATIONSHIP

ROLES OF THE NURSE

- Ensure self-awareness and evaluation of their own beliefs, values, and behaviors.
- Focus on the client's ideas, experiences, and feelings.
- Identify and explore the client's needs and problems. Qᴇᴄᴄ
- Facilitate therapeutic communication.
- Discuss problem-solving alternatives with the client.
- Help to develop the client's strengths and new coping skills.
- Encourage a positive behavior change in the client.
- Assist the client to develop a sense of autonomy and self-reliance.
- Provide education to the client and family about the environment, expectations, disorders, medications, symptom management, and rights of the client.
- Orient the client and family to the care environment, treatments, and expectations regarding safety as well as expected behaviors.
- Establish a welcoming trauma-informed environment.
- Enable health promotion through education.
- Select and advocate for activities that promote participation, recovery and healing.
- Portray genuineness, empathy, and a positive regard toward the client. The nurse practices empathy by remaining nonjudgmental and attempting to understand the client's actions and feelings. This differs from sympathy, which is non-therapeutic, in which the nurse allows oneself to feel the way the client does.

BENEFITS OF THE THERAPEUTIC RELATIONSHIP

Therapeutic relationships contribute to the well-being of those who have a mental illness, as well as other clients, although the treatment goals will be individualized.

- These relationships take time to establish, but even time-limited therapeutic encounters can have positive outcomes.
- Therapeutic relationships have a positive impact on the success of treatment.
- Collaboration with peers and the clinical interdisciplinary team enhances the nurse's ability to examine their own thoughts and feelings, maintain boundaries, and continue to learn from nurse-client relationships.

- Factors that positively affect the development of the therapeutic relationship include
  - NURSE FACTORS
    - Consistent approach to all interaction as therapeutic encounters
    - Adjustment of pace to client's needs
    - Attentive and active listening
    - Positive initial impressions
    - Comfort level during the relationship
    - Self-awareness of own thoughts, values and feelings
    - Consistent availability and follow through
    - Therapeutic use of self in creating a nurse-client alliance
  - CLIENT FACTORS
    - Trusting attitude
    - Willingness to talk
    - Active participation
    - Consistent availability

BOUNDARIES OF THE THERAPEUTIC RELATIONSHIP

Boundaries must be established in order to maintain a safe and professional nurse-client relationship.

- Blurred boundaries occur if the relationship begins to meet the needs of the nurse rather than those of the client, or if the relationship becomes social rather than therapeutic.
  - **Social relationship**: Primary purpose is for socialization or friendship with a focus on the mutual needs of the individuals involved in the relationship.
  - **Therapeutic relationship:** Primary purpose is to identify the client's problems or needs and then focus on assisting the client in meeting or resolving those issues.

The nurse must work to maintain a consistent level of involvement with the client, to reflect on boundary issues frequently, and to maintain awareness of how behaviors can be perceived by others (clients, family members, other health team members).

- **Transference** occurs when the client views a member of the health care team as having characteristics of another person who has been significant to the client's personal life.
  - BEHAVIORS
    - Client expects exclusive services from the nurse, such as extra session time.
    - Client demonstrates jealousy of the nurse's time or attention.
    - Client compares the nurse to a former authority figure.
  - EXAMPLE: A client can see a nurse as being like their parent and thus can demonstrate some of the same behaviors with the nurse that they demonstrated with their parent.
  - NURSING IMPLICATIONS: A nurse should be aware that transference by a client is more likely to occur with a person in authority.

5.1 Phases and tasks of therapeutic relationships

Pre-Orientation

NURSE

Recognize needs of client through review of chart information such as mental and physical examination, client orders or nurse-nurse handoff.

Self-evaluation of personal thoughts concerns, feelings, beliefs and behaviors which may impact client care.

Prepare for tasks required during client care such as review of client medications or scheduled treatments.

Orientation

NURSE

Introduce self to the client and state the purpose of the meetings.

Set the contract: meeting time, place, frequency, duration, and date of termination.

Discuss confidentiality.

Build trust by establishing rapport, expectations, and boundaries.

Set goals with the client.

Explore the client's ideas, issues, and needs.

CLIENT

Meet with the nurse.

Agree to the contract.

Understand the limits of confidentiality.

Understand the expectations and limits of the relationship.

Participate in setting goals.

Begin to explore own thoughts, experiences, and feelings.

Explore the meaning of own behaviors.

Working

NURSE

Maintain relationship according to the contract.

Perform ongoing collection of data to plan and evaluate therapeutic measures.

Facilitate the client's expression of needs and issues.

Encourage the client to problem-solve.

Promote the client's self-esteem.

Foster positive behavioral change.

Explore and deal with resistance and other defense mechanisms.

Recognize transference and countertransference issues.

Re-evaluate the client's problems and goals, and assist with revision of plans as necessary.

Support the client's adaptive alternatives and use of new coping skills.

Remind the client about the date of termination.

CLIENT

Explore problematic areas of life.

Reconsider usual coping behaviors.

Examine own world view and self-concept.

Describe major conflicts and various defenses.

Experience intense feelings and learn to cope with anxiety reactions.

Test new behaviors.

Begin to develop awareness of transference situations.

Try alternative solutions.

Termination

NURSE

Provide opportunity for the client to discuss thoughts and feelings about termination and loss.

Discuss the client's previous experience with separations and loss.

Elicit the client's feelings about the therapeutic work in the nurse-client relationship.

Summarize goals and achievements.

Review memories of work in the sessions.

Express own feelings about sessions to validate the experience with the client.

Discuss ways for the client to incorporate new healthy behaviors into life.

Maintain limits of final termination.

CLIENT

Discuss thoughts and feelings about termination.

Examine previous separation and loss experiences.

Explore the meaning of the therapeutic relationship.

Review goals and achievements.

Discuss plans to continue new behaviors.

Express any feelings of loss related to termination.

Make plans for the future.

Accept termination as final.

5.2 Transference

Transference

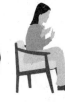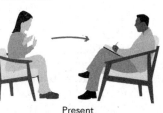

Past   Present

Occurs when the client views a member of the health care team as having characteristics of another person who has been significant to the client's personal life, "This nurse is just like my dad."

5.3 Countertransference

Counter Transference

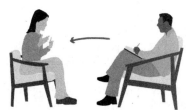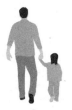

Present   Past

Occurs when a health care team member displaces characteristics of people in their past onto a client. "This client reminds me of my little sister."

- **Countertransference** occurs when a health care team member displaces characteristics of people in their past onto a client.
  - BEHAVIORS
    - Nurse overly identifies with client.
    - Nurse competes with client.
    - Nurse argues with client.
  - EXAMPLE: A nurse can feel defensive and angry with a client for no apparent reason if the client reminds them of a friend who often elicited those feelings.
  - NURSING IMPLICATIONS: A nurse should be aware that clients who induce very strong personal feelings can become objects of countertransference, which interferes with the nurse-client relationship.

Transference

Occurs when the client views a member of the health care team as having characteristics of another person who has been significant to the client's personal life, "This nurse is just like my dad."

Countertransference

Occurs when a health care team member displaces characteristics of people in their past onto a client. "This client reminds me of my little sister."

PHYSICAL SAFETY

- The nurses' station and other areas should be placed to allow for easy observation of clients by staff and access to staff by clients.
- Special safety features (bathroom bars and wheelchair accessibility for clients who are disabled) should be addressed.
- Set up the following provisions to prevent client self-harm or harm by others. Qs
  - No access to sharp or otherwise harmful objects
  - Restriction of client access to restricted or locked areas
  - Monitoring of visitors
  - Restriction of alcohol and illegal substance access or use
  - Restriction of sexual activity among clients
  - Deterrence of elopement from facility
  - Rapid de-escalation of disruptive and potentially violent behaviors through planned interventions by trained staff
- Seclusion rooms and restraints should be set up for safety and used only after all less-restrictive measures have been exhausted. When used, facility policies and procedures must be followed.
- Plan for safe access to recreational areas, occupational therapy, and meeting rooms.

- Reinforce fire, evacuation, and other safety rules to all staff.
  - Provide clear plans for keeping clients and staff safe in emergencies.
  - Maintain staff skills (e.g., cardiopulmonary resuscitation).
- Considerations of room assignments on a 24-hr care unit should include:
  - Personalities of each roommate.
  - The likelihood of nighttime disruptions for a roommate if one client has difficulty sleeping.
  - Mental health and medical diagnoses, such as how two clients who have severe paranoia might interact with each other.

ACTIVITIES WITHIN THE THERAPEUTIC MILIEU

Activities are structured and include time for the following.

- **Community meetings** on the mental health unit should enhance the emotional climate of the therapeutic milieu by promoting: Q EBP
  - Interaction and communication between staff and clients.
  - Decision making skills of clients.
  - A feeling of self-worth among clients.
  - Discussions of common unit objectives (encouraging clients to meet treatment goals and plan for discharge).
  - Discussion of issues of concern to all members of the unit, including common problems, future activities, and the introduction of new clients to the unit.
  - Meetings that can be structured so that they are client-led with decisions made by the group as a whole.
- **Individual therapy** is characterized by scheduled sessions with a mental health provider to address specific mental health concerns (e.g., depression).
- **Group therapy** is characterized by scheduled sessions for a group of clients to address common mental health issues (e.g., substance use disorder).
- **Psychoeducational group**s are based on clients' level of functioning and personal needs (e.g., adverse effects of medication).
- **Recreational activitie**s include games and community outings.
- **Unstructured, flexible time** includes opportunities for the nurse and other staff to observe clients as they interact spontaneously within the milieu.

1. A nurse is talking with a new client who is at risk for suicide following their partner's death. Which of the following statements by the nurse explains the purpose of milieu therapy?

   A. "Milieu therapy is focused on creating a safe, healing, therapeutic environment."

   B. "Milieu therapy is the scheduled activities focused on improved client socialization."

   C. "Milieu therapy consists of scheduled group sessions addressing common mental health needs."

   D. "Milieu therapy's primary focus is on client education based on individual treatment goals."

2. A nurse is discussing the characteristics of a nurse-client relationship with a newly licensed nurse. Which of the following characteristics should the nurse include in the discussion? Select all that apply.

   A. The needs of both participants are met.

   B. An emotional commitment exists between the participants.

   C. All encounters are goal-directed.

   D. Positive behavioral changes are encouraged.

   E. Promotes balance of client autonomy and safety.

3. A nurse is orienting a new client to the activities and therapies on the mental health unit. Match the activity or therapy with the appropriate description.

A. Psychoeducational Groups	1. Scheduled session of all members of mental health unit to enhance and manage the therapeutic milieu.
B. Recreational Therapy	2. Scheduled sessions with a mental health provider to address specific mental health concerns.
C. Group Therapy	3. Scheduled sessions for a group of clients to address common mental health issues
D. Individual Therapy	4. Scheduled sessions focused on use which include socialization with other activities or outings.
E. Community Meeting	5. Scheduled sessions focused on education based on client level of function and needs.

4. A nurse is assisting with planning care for the termination phase of a nurse-client relationship. Which of the following actions should the nurse include in the plan of care?

   A. Discussing ways to use new behaviors

   B. Practicing new problem-solving skills

   C. Developing goals

   D. Establishing boundaries

A nurse is discussing the therapeutic milieu with a newly licensed nurse. Use the ATI Active Learning Template: Basic Concept to complete this item.

UNDERLYING PRINCIPLES: Identify at least five responsibilities of the health care team members to maintain a therapeutic milieu.

NURSING INTERVENTIONS: Identify at least four interventions to prevent client self-harm or harm by others.

Active Learning Scenario Key

Using the ATI Active Learning Template: Basic Concept

UNDERLYING PRINCIPLES
- Promote independence for self-care and individual growth.
- Treat clients as individuals.
- Allow choices for clients within the daily routine and treatment plan.
- Apply rules of fair treatment for all clients.
- Model good social behavior.
- Work cooperatively as a team to provide care.
- Maintain professional boundaries with clients.
- Maintain a professional appearance and demeanor.
- Promote safe and satisfying peer interactions among clients.
- Practice open communication techniques with health team members and clients.
- Promote positive feelings of self-worth and hope for the future.

NURSING INTERVENTIONS
- Prevent access to sharp or harmful objects.
- Inhibit client access to restricted or locked areas.
- Monitor visitors.
- Restrict access to alcohol and illegal substance use.
- Restrict sexual activity with other clients.
- Deter elopement from facility.
- Provide rapid de-escalation of disruptive and potentially violent behaviors.
- Be aware of facility policies and procedures for seclusion or restraints.
- Provide safe access to recreational areas, therapy areas, and meeting rooms.

Ⓝ *NCLEX® Connection: Psychosocial Integrity, Therapeutic Environment*

Application Exercises Key

1. A. **CORRECT:** When taking action and discussing the purpose of milieu therapy, the nurse should include that the primary purpose is to create and maintain a safe, healing, therapeutic environment. Recreation therapy and activities may be used in client care and treatment plans and is focused on improving client socialization. Group therapy involves scheduled sessions which address common client needs. Psychoeducational groups focus on education based on the client needs and levels of functioning.

Ⓝ *NCLEX® Connection: Psychosocial Integrity, Therapeutic Communication*

2. C, D, E. **CORRECT:** A therapeutic nurse-client relationship focuses on the needs of the client. Establishes a therapeutic alliance which are therapeutic rather than based on an emotional commitment between the participants. Emotional commitment between individuals is characteristic of an intimate or social relationship, rather than one that is therapeutic. Therapeutic nurse-client relationships are characterized as being goal-directed, encouraging positive behavioral change and assists clients in developing autonomy and balances this with client safety.

Ⓝ *NCLEX® Connection: Psychosocial Integrity, Therapeutic Environment*

3. A, 5; B, 4; C, 3; D, 2; E, 1

Therapeutic milieu includes activities, therapies and groups which focus on improving client mental health and well-being, a sense of security and promotes recovery.

Ⓝ *NCLEX® Connection: Psychosocial Integrity, Therapeutic Environment*

4. A. **CORRECT:** When assisting generating solutions, the nurse should discuss ways for the client to incorporate new healthy behaviors into life is an appropriate task for the termination phase. Practicing new problem-solving skills is an appropriate task for the working phase. Developing goals and establishing boundaries are appropriate tasks for the orientation phase.

Ⓝ *NCLEX® Connection: Psychosocial Integrity, Behavioral Management*

CHAPTER 6 Diverse Practice Settings

Mental health nursing occurs in acute care and community settings, as well as in forensic nursing settings.

In all settings, nurses are advocates for clients who have mental illness. Referral of clients and their families to organizations and agencies that provide additional resources can provide significant support to individuals.

For example, the National Alliance on Mental Illness (NAMI) is a grassroots organization with the goals of improving the quality of life for persons with mental illness and providing research to better treat or eradicate mental illness. For more information, visit the NAMI website. Qᴛᴄ

SETTINGS FOR MENTAL HEALTH CARE

ACUTE CARE

This setting provides intensive treatment and supervision in locked units for clients who are in an emotional crisis and present a danger to self or others.
- Care in these facilities helps stabilize mental illness manifestations and promotes the clients' rapid return to the community.
- Staff is made up of an interprofessional team with management provided by nurses developing individualized plans that are client- and family-centered. Facilities might be privately owned or general hospitals, with payment provided by private funds or insurance. Qᴛᴄ
- Facilities also might be state owned, with much of the funding provided for homeless clients. State-run facilities also often provide full-time acute care for forensic clients (those in a correctional setting) who have severe mental illness.
- Case management programs assist with client transition to a community setting after discharge from the acute care facility.

COMMUNITY

Primary care is provided in community-based settings, which include clinics, schools and day-care centers, partial hospitalization programs, substance treatment facilities, forensic settings, psychosocial rehabilitation programs, telephone crisis counseling centers, and home health care.
- Nurses working in community care programs help to stabilize or improve clients' mental functioning within a community. They also assist with teaching, support, and make referrals in order to promote positive social activities.
- Nursing interventions in community settings provide for primary treatment as well as primary, secondary, and tertiary prevention of mental illness.

FORENSIC NURSING

Forensic nursing is a combination of biophysical education and forensic science. It is the utilization of nursing science to public or legal proceedings. The registered nurses use scientific investigation, collection of evidence, analysis, prevention, and treatment of trauma and/or death of perpetrators and victims of violence, abuse, and traumatic accidents.

REHABILITATION

This setting provides a structured environment where clients may focus on cognitive and behavioral changes related to substance use, non-suicidal self-injury, eating disorders, and other anxiety related disorders.
- Clients may require assistance with activities of daily living, like adhering to a medication regimen, eating, and daily hygiene.
- Treatment typically lasts from weeks to months.

HISTORY OF MENTAL HEALTH CARE IN THE UNITED STATES

- Most clients who have severe mental illness were treated solely in acute care facilities before the middle of the twentieth century.
- Congress passed a series of acts in 1946, 1955, and 1963 in response to the appalling condition of facilities for the mentally ill. This began a trend to deinstitutionalize mental health care.
- Clients who had lived in acute care mental health facilities for many years were discharged into the community at a time when community mental health facilities were often unprepared to deal with this influx.
- The concept of case management was introduced around 1970 to meet the individual needs of clients in a mental health setting.
- Managed care through health maintenance organizations (HMOs), preferred provider organizations (PPOs), and others began limiting hospital stays for clients in a general medical setting starting around 1980.

- In 1999, mental illness was defined as a disability in the Americans with Disabilities Act, stating those individuals with mental illnesses had a right to live in the community.
- Managed Behavioral Healthcare Organizations (MBHOs) were later developed to coordinate care and limit stays in acute care facilities for clients needing mental health care.
- This began the trend to develop a continuum of acute care facilities and community mental health facilities to provide for all levels of behavioral health care needs.
- Complete and accurate documentation of client needs and progress by nurses and other health care professionals is needed to ensure quality care for each client. Qᴸ
- Factors that will affect the future of mental health care include the following.
  - An increase in the aging population
  - An increase in cultural diversity within the United States
  - The expansion of technology, which might provide new settings for client care, as well as new ways to treat mental illness more effectively

CLIENT CARE

Nursing role

Nurses in acute care mental health facilities use the nursing process and a holistic approach to provide care. Nursing roles include the following:
- Overall management of the unit, including client activities and therapeutic milieu
- Ensuring safe administration and monitoring of all client medications
- Implementation of individualized client treatment plans, including assisting with client teaching
- Documentation of the nursing process for each client
- Managing crises as they arise
- A case manager helps the client to coordinate their mental health treatment, such as medications, appointments, or arrange transportation.

Interprofessional team members

- Team members in acute care include nurses, mental health workers (who perform duties similar to assistive personnel in other health care facilities), psychologists, psychiatrists, other general health care providers, social workers, counselors, occupational and other specialty therapists, and pharmacists. Qᴛᴄ
- The interprofessional team has the primary responsibility of planning and monitoring individualized treatment plans or clinical pathways of care, depending on the philosophy and policy of the facility.
- Plans for discharge to home or to a community facility begin from the time of admission and continue with the implementation of the initial treatment plan or clinical pathway.

ACUTE MENTAL HEALTH CARE SETTINGS

- Criteria to justify admission to an acute care facility include. Qᴛᴄ
  - A clear risk of the client's danger to self or others
  - An inability to meet own basic needs
  - Failure to meet expected outcomes of community-based treatment
  - A dangerous decline in the mental health status of a client undergoing long-term treatment
  - A client having a medical need in addition to a mental illness
- Goals of acute mental health treatment include the following.
  - Prevention of the client harming self or others
  - Stabilizing mental health crises
  - Return of clients who are severally ill to some type of community care

COMMUNITY HEALTH SETTINGS

- Nurses play a vital role in linking acute care facilities with community care facilities.
- Intensive outpatient programs promote community reintegration for clients.
- Mobile crisis teams are specially trained mental health professionals who provide emergency psychiatric care on-site of the client's location.

TELEHEALTH

- The role of telehealth services for client mental health care has expanded to meet the needs of those who cannot attend typical in-person treatment.
- Many clients who use telehealth as their primary means of receiving treatment.
- Insurance companies have expanded their coverage to include reimbursement for telehealth services.
- Client's may receive telehealth services from a variety of members of the interprofessional team.

Levels of prevention

Three levels of prevention are used by nurses when implementing community care interventions/instructing. Qᴛᴄ

Primary prevention promotes health and emphasizes efforts on preventing mental health problems from occurring.

> Example: A nurse instructs a community education program on stress reduction techniques.

Secondary prevention focuses on early detection of mental illness.

> Example: A nurse screens older adults in the community for depression.

Tertiary prevention focuses on rehabilitation and prevention of further problems in clients who have previous diagnoses. Mental illness is present and with tertiary prevention, the goal is to prevent further deterioration or complications.

> Example: A nurse leads a support group for clients who have completed a substance use disorder program.

Community-based mental health programs

Community-based mental health programs are a continuum of mental health agencies with varying treatment intensity levels to allow clients to remain safe in the least restrictive environment possible.

Partial hospitalization programs
- These programs provide intense short-term treatment for clients who are well enough to go home every night and who have a responsible person at home to provide support and a safe environment.
- Certain detoxification programs are a specialized form of partial hospitalization for clients who require medical supervision, stress management, substance use disorder counseling, and relapse prevention.

Assertive community treatment (ACT)
- This includes nontraditional case management and treatment by an interprofessional team for clients who have severe manifestations of mental illness and are nonadherent with traditional treatment.
- ACT helps to reduce recurrences of hospitalizations and provides crisis intervention, assistance with independent living, and information regarding resources for necessary support services. ACT teams work with clients in their homes and in agencies, hospitals, and clinics.

Community mental health centers
These facilities provide a variety of services for a wide range of community clients, including:
- Educational groups
- Medication dispensing programs
- Individual and family counseling programs

Psychosocial rehabilitation programs
These programs provide a structured range of programs for clients in a mental health setting, including:
- Residential services
- Day programs for older adults

Home based services: Home based services provide mental health assessment, interventions, and family support in the client's home. This is implemented most often for children, older adults, and clients who have medical conditions. With psychiatric home care, there are four criteria that must be met. The client must be homebound, have a psychiatric diagnosis, need the skills of a mental health nurse, and a plan of care developed by the health care provider.

ROLES OF NURSES IN DIVERSE MENTAL HEALTH PRACTICE SETTINGS

REGISTERED NURSE

- Educational preparation: diploma, associate degree, or baccalaureate degree in nursing, with additional on-the-job training and continuing education in mental health care
- Can work in either an acute care or community-based facility
- Functions within a facility using the nursing process to provide care and treatment (medication)
- Manages care for a group of clients within a unit of the facility

ADVANCED PRACTICE NURSE

- Educational preparation: advanced nursing degree in behavioral health (master's degree, doctorate, nurse practitioner, or clinical nurse specialist)
- Can work independently, often supervising individuals or groups in either an acute care or community-based setting
- Can have prescription privileges, provide various types of therapy, and is able to independently recommend interventions
- Can manage and administrate the care for an entire facility
- Can lead research and quality improvement efforts

1. A nurse is working in a community mental health facility. Which of the following services does this type of program provide? (Select all that apply.)

   A. Educational groups

   B. Medication dispensing programs

   C. Individual counseling programs

   D. Detoxification programs

   E. Family therapy

2. A nurse is assisting with planning care for several clients who are attending community-based mental health programs. Which of the following clients should the nurse visit first?

   A. A client who reports feeling decreased self esteem.

   B. A client who requests a change of antipsychotic medication due to some new adverse effects.

   C. A client who reports hearing a voice saying that life is not worth living anymore.

   D. A client who tells the nurse about experiencing manifestations of severe anxiety before and during a job interview.

3. A nurse in an acute mental health facility is assisting with discharge planning for a client who has a severe mental illness and requires supervision. The client's partner works all day but is home by late afternoon. Which of the following strategies should the nurse suggest for follow-up care?

   A. Receiving daily care from a home health aide

   B. Having a weekly visit from a nurse case worker

   C. Attending a partial hospitalization program

   D. Visiting a community mental health center on a daily basis

4. A community mental health nurse is assisting in planning care to address the issue of depression among older adult clients in the community. Which of the following interventions should the nurse implement as a method of tertiary prevention?

   A. Educating clients on health promotion techniques to reduce the risk of depression.

   B. Performing screenings for depression at community health programs.

   C. Establishing rehabilitation programs to decrease the effects of depression.

   D. Providing support groups for clients at risk for depression.

5. A nurse is caring for a group of clients. Which of the following clients should a nurse consider for referral to an assertive community treatment (ACT) group?

   A. A client in an acute care mental health facility who has fallen several times while running down the hallway.

   B. A client who lives at home and keeps "forgetting" to come in for a scheduled monthly antipsychotic injection for schizophrenia.

   C. A client in a day treatment program who reports increasing anxiety during group therapy.

   D. A client in a weekly grief support group who reports still missing a deceased partner who has been dead for 3 months.

Active Learning Scenario

A nurse is assisting with an in-service program regarding acute mental health treatment for a group of newly licensed nurses. What should the nurse recommend for inclusion in this presentation? Use the ATI Active Learning Template: Basic Concept to complete this item.

RELATED CONTENT: Identify two criteria for admitting a client to a mental health facility.

UNDERLYING PRINCIPLES: Describe two concepts of mental health treatment.

NURSING INTERVENTIONS: Describe two interventions that apply to acute mental health care.

Application Exercises Key

1. A, B, C, E. **CORRECT:** The nurse is aware that community mental health facilities offer the following services which include educational groups, medication dispensing programs, individual counseling programs, and family therapy. Detoxification programs are services provided in a partial hospitalization program.

   Ⓝ *NCLEX® Connection: Psychosocial Integrity, Therapeutic Environment*

2. C. **CORRECT:** A client who hears a voice saying life is not worth living anymore is at greatest risk for self-harm, and the nurse should visit this client first. Although the other clients have health care needs, the client with a safety risk is highest priority.

   Ⓝ *NCLEX® Connection: Coordinated Care, Establishing Priorities*

3. C. **CORRECT:** When taking action, the nurse should suggest the following strategy for follow-up care for a client who has a severe mental illness and requires supervision: a partial hospitalization program can provide treatment during the day while allowing the client to spend nights at home, as long as a responsible family member is present. Daily care provided by a home health aide, weekly visit from a case worker, and daily visits to a community mental health center will not provide consistent supervision for this client.

   Ⓝ *NCLEX® Connection: Psychosocial Integrity, Mental Health Concepts*

4. C. **CORRECT:** Rehabilitation programs are an example of tertiary prevention. Tertiary prevention deals with prevention of further problems in clients already diagnosed with mental illness. Educating and providing support for risks is considered a primary prevention intervention. Screenings are considered a secondary prevention intervention.

   Ⓝ *NCLEX® Connection: Psychosocial Integrity, Mental Health Concepts*

5. B. **CORRECT:** An ACT group works with clients who are nonadherent with traditional therapy (the client in a home setting who keeps "forgetting" a scheduled injection). A client in acute care who has been running and falling should be helped by the treatment team on the client's unit. A client who has anxiety might be referred to a counselor or mental health provider. A client who is grieving for a deceased partner who died 3 months ago is currently involved in an appropriate intervention.

   Ⓝ *NCLEX® Connection: Coordinated Care, Referral Process*

Active Learning Scenario Key

Using the ATI Active Learning Template: Basic Concept

RELATED CONTENT
- Clear risk of the client's danger to self and others.
- Failure to meet expected outcomes of community-based treatment.
- A dangerous decline in the mental health status of a client undergoing long-term treatment
- A client having a medical need in addition to a mental illness.

UNDERLYING PRINCIPLES
- Goals of acute mental health treatment:
  - Prevention of the client harming self or others
  - Stabilizing mental health crises
  - Return of clients who are severally ill to some type of community care
- Interprofessional team members in acute care include nurses, mental health technicians, psychologists, psychiatrists, other general health care providers, social workers, counselors, occupational and other specialty therapists, and pharmacists.

NURSING INTERVENTIONS
- **Who:** The interprofessional team member's primary responsibility is planning and monitoring individualized treatment plans or clinical pathways of care.
- **When:** Assisting with plans for discharge to home or to a community facility begin from the time of admission.
- **How:** Nursing roles include assisting with the overall management of the unit, including client activities and therapeutic milieu.
- Ensuring safe administration and monitoring of client medications.
- Assist with the implementation of individualized client treatment plans, including reinforcement of client teaching.
- Documentation of the nursing process for each client.
- Assisting with managing crises as they arise.

Ⓝ *NCLEX® Connection: Coordinated Care, Collaboration with Multidisciplinary Team*

When reviewing the following chapters, keep in mind the relevant topics and tasks of the NCLEX outline.

Psychosocial Integrity

BEHAVIORAL MANAGEMENT: Participate in client group session.

COPING MECHANISMS: Recognize abilities of client to adapt to temporary/permanent role changes.

MENTAL HEALTH CONCEPTS: Recognize client use of defense mechanisms.

STRESS MANAGEMENT: Implement measures to reduce environmental stressors.

SUPPORT SYSTEMS: Identify client support systems/resources.

THERAPEUTIC COMMUNICATION
Provide emotional support to client.

Encourage client-appropriate use of verbal and nonverbal communication.

Reduction of Risk Potential

POTENTIAL FOR COMPLICATIONS OF DIAGNOSTIC TESTS/ TREATMENTS/PROCEDURES
Provide care for client receiving electroconvulsive therapy (ECT).

Identify client risk, and implement interventions.

CHAPTER 7

Psychoanalysis, Psychotherapy, and Behavioral Therapies

Psychoanalysis, psychotherapy, and behavioral therapies are approaches to addressing mental health issues using various methods and theoretical bases.

Nursing responsibilities can vary based on the type of therapy. Often the nurse will not be performing the therapy, but rather collecting initial assessment data, recognizing the client's need for therapy, evaluating manifestation and treatment progression, or even advocating for the client's right to treatment. Nurses being aware and familiar with the different types of therapy helps support the client as they engage in the therapy.

The nurse can reinforce education to the client on the benefits of the different types of therapies and what types of diagnoses they can assist with.

PSYCHOANALYSIS

Classical psychoanalysis is a therapeutic process of assessing unconscious thoughts and feelings, and resolving conflict by talking to a psychoanalyst. Clients attend many sessions over the course of months to years.

- Due to the length of psychoanalytic therapy and health insurance constraints, classical psychoanalysis is unlikely to be the sole therapy of choice.
- Psychoanalysis was first developed by Sigmund Freud to resolve internal conflicts which, he contended, always occur from early childhood experiences. Psychoanalysis, as developed by Freud, is seldom used today.
- Past relationships are a common focus for therapy and to uncover unconscious conflicts.

Transference, which includes feelings that the client has developed toward the therapist in relation to similar feelings toward significant persons in the client's early childhood

Countertransference, the unconscious feelings that the healthcare worker has toward the client. The client can remind them of a person from their past in a positive or negative manner.

THERAPEUTIC TOOLS

Free association, which is the spontaneous, uncensored verbalization of whatever comes to a client's mind

Dream analysis and interpretation, believed by Freud to be urges and impulses of the unconscious mind that played out through the dreams of clients

Use of **defense mechanisms** can help decrease or prevent anxiety by blocking awareness of negative feelings.

PSYCHOTHERAPY

Psychotherapy involves more verbal therapist-to-client interaction than classic psychoanalysis. The client and the therapist develop a trusting relationship to explore the client's issues and can take 20 or more sessions.

Psychodynamic psychotherapy employs the same tools as psychoanalysis, but it focuses more on the client's present state, rather than their early life. This type of therapy tends to last longer than other treatment approaches.

Interpersonal psychotherapy (IPT) assists clients in addressing specific issues. It can improve interpersonal relationships, communication, role-relationship, and bereavement. The premise with interpersonal therapy is that many mental health disorders are influenced by interpersonal interactions and the social context. The goal is to improve interpersonal and social functioning which will reduce the psychiatric manifestations.

Cognitive therapy is based on the cognitive model, which focuses on individual thoughts and behaviors to solve current issues. The belief is that thoughts come before feelings and actions. It treats depression, anxiety, eating disorders, and other issues that can improve by changing a client's attitude toward life experiences.

Behavioral therapy
- In protest of Freud's psychoanalytic theory, behavioral theorists (Ivan Pavlov, John B. Watson, and B.F. Skinner) felt that changing behavior was the key to treating problems (anxiety or depressive disorders).
- Behavioral therapy is based on the theory that behavior is learned and has consequences. Abnormal behavior results from an attempt to avoid painful feelings. Changing abnormal or maladaptive behavior can occur without the need for insight into the underlying cause of the behavior.
- Behavioral therapies teach clients ways to decrease anxiety or avoidant behavior and give clients an opportunity to practice techniques. Behavioral therapy teaches activities to help the client reduce anxious and avoidant behavior like relaxation training and modeling.
- Behavioral therapy has been used successfully to treat clients who have phobias, substance use or addictive disorders, and other issues.

Eye movement desensitization reprocessing (EMDR) is a focused approach that encourages the client to reconnect traumatizing memories and emotions in a safe structured environment that allows the client to reprocess their emotions and feelings through the use of adaptive defense mechanisms. EMDR is effective in treating anxiety and trauma related disorders.

Cognitive-behavioral therapy uses both cognitive and behavioral approaches to assist a client with anxiety management. This therapy takes into account what clients think influences their feelings and behaviors.

Dialectical behavior therapy is a cognitive-behavioral therapy for clients who have a personality disorder and exhibit self-injurious behavior. This therapy focuses on gradual behavior changes and provides acceptance and validation for these clients.

USE OF COGNITIVE THERAPY

Cognitive reframing

Changing cognitive distortions can decrease anxiety. Cognitive reframing assists clients to identify negative thoughts that produce anxiety, examine the cause, and develop supportive ideas that replace negative self-talk. For example, a client who has a depressive disorder might say they are "a bad person" who has "never done anything good" in their life. Through therapy, this client can change their thinking to realize that they might have made some bad choices, but that they are not "a bad person."

Priority restructuring: Assists clients to identify what requires priority (devoting energy to pleasurable activities).

Journal keeping: Helps clients write down stressful thoughts and has a positive effect on well-being.

Assertiveness training: Teaches clients to express feelings, and solve problems in a nonaggressive manner.

Monitoring thoughts: Helps clients to be aware of negative thinking.

TYPES AND USES OF BEHAVIORAL THERAPY

Modeling

A therapist or others serve as role models for a client, who imitates this modeling to improve behavior.

USE IN MENTAL HEALTH NURSING: Modeling can occur in the acute care milieu to help clients improve interpersonal skills. The therapist demonstrates appropriate behavior in a stressful situation with the goal of having the client imitate the behavior.

Operant conditioning

The client receives positive rewards for positive behavior (positive reinforcement).

USE IN MENTAL HEALTH NURSING: As an example: a client receives tokens for good behavior, and they can exchange them for a privilege or other items.

Systematic desensitization

This therapy is the planned, progressive, or graduated exposure to anxiety-provoking stimuli in real-life situations, or by imagining events that cause anxiety. During exposure, the client uses relaxation techniques to suppress anxiety response.

USE IN MENTAL HEALTH NURSING: Systematic desensitization begins with the client mastering relaxation techniques. Then, the client is exposed to increasing levels of the anxiety-producing stimulus (either imagined or real) and uses relaxation to overcome anxiety. The client is then able to tolerate a greater and greater level of the stimulus until anxiety no longer interferes with functioning. Used to assist clients who have phobias that are anxiety producing.

Aversion therapy

Pairing of a maladaptive behavior with a punishment or unpleasant stimuli to promote a change in the behavior.

USE IN MENTAL HEALTH NURSING: A therapist or treatment team can use unpleasant stimuli (bitter taste, mild electric shock), as punishment for behaviors (alcohol use disorder, violence, self-mutilation, and thumb-sucking). With aversion therapy, ongoing supervision and evaluation is essential for those administering the aversion therapy.

Meditation, guided imagery, diaphragmatic breathing, muscle relaxation, and biofeedback

This therapy uses various techniques to control pain, tension, and anxiety.

USE IN MENTAL HEALTH NURSING: A nurse can reinforce how to perform diaphragmatic breathing to a client having a panic attack, or to a female client in labor.

OTHER TECHNIQUES

Flooding: Exposing a client, while in the company of a therapist, to a great deal of an undesirable stimulus in an attempt to turn off the anxiety response

Response prevention: Preventing a client from performing a compulsive behavior with the intent that anxiety will diminish

Thought stopping: Teaching a client, when negative thoughts or compulsive behaviors arise, to say or shout, "stop," and substitute a positive thought. The goal over time is for the client to use the command silently.

Trauma focused CBT: The treatment approach often begins with psychoeducation about trauma responses and coping mechanisms. Gradual exposure to trauma memory as a way to "redo" the trauma experience in a more adaptive way.

Validation therapy: Useful for clients with neurocognitive disorders. It is a process of communication with a disoriented older adult client by respecting and validating their feelings in a time or place that is real to them, even though it does not relate to actual reality.

Virtual reality exposure therapy: Clients are placed into a virtual controlled environment where the therapist, in-person or remote, can help alleviate depression, anxiety, phobias, post-traumatic stress disorder, and attachment issues.

Active Learning Scenario

A nurse working in an acute mental health unit is caring for a client who has a personality disorder. The client refuses to attend group meetings and will not speak to other clients or attend unit activities. The client enjoys visiting with staff and requests daily to take a walk outside with a staff member. The provider prescribes behavioral therapy with operant conditioning. Use the ATI Active Learning Template: Therapeutic Procedure to complete this item.

DESCRIPTION OF PROCEDURE: Discuss behavioral therapy and operant conditioning.

OUTCOMES/EVALUATION: Identify an appropriate client outcome.

NURSING INTERVENTIONS: Identify an appropriate nursing action to implement operant conditioning with this client.

Application Exercises

1. A nurse is reinforcing teaching about free association as a therapeutic tool with a client who has major depressive disorder. Which of the following client statements indicates understanding of this technique?
   A. "Even if my anxiety improves, I will need to continue this therapy for 6 weeks."
   B. "The therapist will focus on my past relationships during our sessions."
   C. "Psychoanalysis will help me reduce my anxiety by changing my behaviors."
   D. "This therapy will address my conscious feelings about stressful experiences."

2. A nurse is discussing free association as a therapeutic tool with a client who has major depressive disorder. Which of the following client statements indicates understanding of this technique?
   A. "I will write down my dreams as soon as I wake up."
   B. "I might begin to associate my therapist with important people in my life."
   C. "I can learn to express myself in a nonaggressive manner."
   D. "I should say the first thing that comes to my mind."

3. A nurse is assisting with planning cognitive reframing techniques for a client who has an anxiety disorder. Which of the following techniques should the nurse recommend to include in the plan of care? (Select all that apply.)
   A. Priority restructuring
   B. Monitoring thoughts
   C. Diaphragmatic breathing
   D. Journal keeping
   E. Meditation

4. A nurse is caring for a client who has a new prescription for disulfiram for treatment of alcohol use disorder. The nurse informs the client that this medication can cause nausea and vomiting when alcohol is consumed. Which of the following types of treatment is this method an example?
   A. Aversion therapy
   B. Flooding
   C. Biofeedback
   D. Dialectical behavior therapy

5. A nurse is assisting with systematic desensitization for a client who has an extreme fear of elevators. Which of the following actions should the nurse implement with this form of therapy?
   A. Demonstrate riding in an elevator, and then ask the client to imitate the behavior.
   B. Advise the client to say "stop" out loud every time they begin to feel an anxiety response related to an elevator.
   C. Gradually expose the client to an elevator while practicing relaxation techniques.
   D. Stay with the client in an elevator until the anxiety response diminishes.

Active Learning Scenario Key

Using the ATI Active Learning Template: Therapeutic Procedure

DESCRIPTION OF PROCEDURE
- Behavioral therapy is based on the theory that behavior is learned and has consequences. These therapies teach clients ways to decrease anxiety or avoidant behavior and give clients an opportunity to practice techniques.
- Operant conditioning provides the client with positive rewards for positive behavior.

OUTCOMES/EVALUATION
- The client will attend group meetings.
- The client will attend unit activities.
- The client will appropriately socialize with other clients on the unit.

NURSING INTERVENTIONS
- The nurse will use tokens, or something similar, to reward the client for a positive change in behavior. The client can use these tokens for larger rewards (a walk outside with a staff member).
- The nurse will provide positive feedback and encouragement for a positive change in behavior.

Ⓝ *NCLEX® Connection: Psychosocial Integrity, Behavioral Management*

Application Exercises Key

1. B. **CORRECT:** When evaluating a form of therapy for anxiety disorder, the nurse should identify that classical psychoanalysis is a therapeutic process that requires many sessions over months to years and places a common focus on past relationships to identify the cause of the anxiety disorder. Classical psychoanalysis focuses on identifying and resolving the cause of the anxiety rather than changing behavior. Classical psychoanalysis assesses unconscious, rather than conscious, thoughts and feelings.

   Ⓝ *NCLEX® Connection: Psychosocial Integrity, Coping Mechanisms*

2. D. **CORRECT:** When taking action, the nurse should identify that free association is the spontaneous, uncensored verbalization of whatever comes to a client's mind. Dream analysis and interpretation are therapeutic tools. However, they are not an example of free association. Associating the therapist with significant persons in the client's life is an example of transference rather than free association. Learning to express feelings and solve problems in a nonaggressive manner is an example of assertiveness training, rather than free association.

   Ⓝ *NCLEX® Connection: Psychosocial Integrity, Behavioral Management*

3. A, B, D. **CORRECT:** When planning care for a client who has anxiety disorder the nurse should identify and use priority restructuring, journaling, and monitoring thoughts is cognitive reframing techniques. Diaphragmatic breathing is a form of behavioral therapy rather than a cognitive reframing technique. Meditation is a form of behavioral therapy rather than a cognitive reframing technique.

   Ⓝ *NCLEX® Connection: Psychosocial Integrity, Behavioral Interventions*

4. A. **CORRECT:** The nurse should identify that aversion therapy pairs a maladaptive behavior with unpleasant stimuli to promote a change in behavior and is used for a client who has a new prescription for disulfiram for treatment of alcohol use disorder. Flooding is planned exposure to an undesirable stimulus in an attempt to turn off the anxiety response. Biofeedback is a behavioral therapy to control pain, tension, and anxiety. Dialectical behavior therapy is a cognitive-behavioral therapy for clients who have a personality disorder and exhibit self-injurious behavior.

   Ⓝ *NCLEX® Connection: Psychosocial Integrity, Chemical and Other Dependencies/Substance Use Disorder*

5. C. **CORRECT:** Demonstration followed by client imitation of the behavior is an example of modeling. Instructing a client to say "stop" when anxiety occurs is an example of thought stopping. Systematic desensitization is the planned, progressive exposure to anxiety-provoking stimuli. During this exposure, relaxation techniques suppress the anxiety response. Exposing the client to a great deal of an undesirable stimulus in an attempt to turn off the anxiety response is an example of flooding.

   Ⓝ *NCLEX® Connection: Psychosocial Integrity, Behavioral Management*

CHAPTER 8

UNIT 2 TRADITIONAL NONPHARMACOLOGICAL THERAPIES

CHAPTER 8 ## Group and Family Therapy

Therapy is an intensive treatment that involves open therapeutic communication with participants who are willing to take part in therapy. Although individual therapy is an important treatment for mental illness, group and family therapies are also a part of the treatment plan for many clients in a mental health setting.

Leaders guide group and family therapy, and they can employ various leadership styles. Democratic leadership supports group interaction and decision making to solve problems. In group settings, more than one client can be involved. Therapy groups offer each client opportunities for growth and a feeling of belonging. Laissez-faire leadership progresses without any attempt by the leader to control the direction. In autocratic leadership, the leader completely controls the direction and structure of the group without allowing group interaction or decision making to solve problems.

Examples of group therapy topics include stress management, substance use disorders, medication education, understanding mental illness, and dual diagnoses.

Group therapy

Group process is the verbal and nonverbal communication that occurs during group sessions, including how the work progresses and how members interact with one another.

Group norm is the way the group behaves during sessions and, over time, it provides structure for the group. For example, a group norm could be that members raise their hand to be recognized by the leader before they speak. Another norm could be that all members sit in the same places for each session.

Hidden agenda: Some group members (or the leader) might have goals different from the stated group goals that can disrupt group processes. For example, three members might try to embarrass another member whom they dislike.

The **dynamics** of a group are affected by the group either being open or closed.

GROUP MEMBERSHIP

- A **homogeneous** group is one in which all members share a certain chosen characteristic (e.g., diagnosis or gender). Membership of heterogeneous groups is not based on a shared chosen personal characteristic. An example of a heterogeneous group is all clients on a unit, including a mixture of men and women who have a wide range of diagnoses.
- A **subgroup** is a small number of people within a larger group who function separately from the group.
- Groups can be open (new members join as old members leave) or closed (no new members join after formation of the group).

8.1 Focus and goals for individual, family, and group therapies

Individual	*Family*	*Group*
FOCUS	FOCUS	FOCUS
Client needs and problems	Family needs and problems within family dynamics	Helping individuals develop more functional and satisfying relations within a group setting
The therapeutic relationship	Improving family functioning	
GOALS	GOALS	GOALS
Make more positive individual decisions.	Learn effective ways for dealing with mental illness within the family.	Goals vary depending on type of group, but clients generally:
Make productive life decisions.	Improve understanding among family members.	Discover that members share some common feelings, experiences, and thoughts.
Develop a strong sense of self.	Maximize positive interaction among family members.	Experience positive behavior changes as a result of group interaction and feedback.

COMPONENTS OF THERAPY SESSIONS

- Use of open and clear communication
- Cohesiveness and guidelines for the therapy session
- Direction toward a particular goal
- Opportunities for development of interpersonal skills, resolution of personal and family issues, and development of appropriate, satisfying relationships.
- Encouragement of the client to maximize positive interactions, feel empowered to make decisions, and strengthen feelings of self-worth
- Communication regarding respect among all members
- Support, as well as education regarding support topics (e.g., available community resources for support)

GROUP THERAPY GOALS

- Sharing common feelings and concerns
- Sharing stories and experiences
- Diminishing feelings of isolation
- Creating a community of healing and restoration
- Providing a more cost-effective environment than that of individual therapy

CONCERNS

- Privacy
- Not all members may receive equal attention.
- Personal opinions may be discouraged by group norms.
- Disruptive members can decrease a group's effectiveness.

AGE GROUPS IN GROUP THERAPY

Children: Group therapy may be in the form of play while talking about a common experience.

Adolescent: Group therapy is especially valuable, as this age group typically has strong peer relationships. Qpcc

Older adult: Group therapy helps with socialization and sharing of memories.

PHASES OF GROUP DEVELOPMENT

Planning phase

PRIMARY FOCUS: Identify group characteristics like member inclusion, group name, seating configuration, and group schedule.

RESPONSIBILITIES
- Consider group composition. For example, a client who is withdrawn may not interact well with a client who tends to probe other members.
- An overcrowded room may cause discomfort and anxiety while a large room for a small group does not encourage intimacy.
- A circular seating configuration emphasizes equality, especially when choosing a democratic leadership style.

Orientation phase

PRIMARY FOCUS: Define the purpose and goals of the group.

RESPONSIBILITIES
- The group leader sets a tone of respect, trust, and confidentiality among members. The group leader is active and provides the purpose of the group.
- Members get to know each other and the group leader.
- There is a discussion about termination.

Working phase

PRIMARY FOCUS: Promote problem-solving skills to facilitate behavioral changes. Power and control issues can dominate in this phase.

RESPONSIBILITIES
- The group leader uses therapeutic communication to encourage group work toward meeting goals.
- Members take informal roles within the group, which can interfere with, or favor, group progress toward goals.
- Cohesiveness has been established and the role of the leader is gradually diminishing.

Termination phase

PRIMARY FOCUS: This marks the end of group sessions.

RESPONSIBILITIES
- Group members discuss termination issues.
- The leader summarizes the work of the group and individual contributions.
- Members of a group can take on any of a number of roles.
- Feedback regarding the group therapy is elicited.

ROLES

Maintenance roles: Members who take on these roles tend to help maintain the purpose and process of the group. For example, the harmonizer attempts to prevent conflict in the group.

Task roles: Members take on various tasks within the group process. An example is the recorder, who takes notes and records what occurs during each session.

Individual roles: These roles tend to prevent teamwork, because individuals take on roles to promote their own agenda. Examples include the dominator, who tries to control other members, and the recognition seeker, who boasts about personal achievements.

GROUP CHARACTERISTICS

Characteristics can vary depending on the health care setting.

Acute mental health setting: Members can vary on a daily basis, and the focus of the group is on relief. Unit activities will directly impact the group, and the leader must provide a higher level of structure.

Outpatient setting: Members are often consistent, the focus of the group is on growth, external influences are limited, and the leader can allow members an opportunity in determining the group's direction.

Virtual groups: Members meet remotely through teleconferencing technologies. This is ideal for members who have limited transportation resources or live in rural areas. Some challenges of virtual groups are difficulties reading nonverbal cues of communication, losing control of group settings, and a lack of full presence.

Families and family therapy

TYPES OF FAMILIES

Nuclear families include children who reside with married parents

Single-parent families include children who live with a single adult that can be related or nonrelated to the children

Adoptive families include children who live with parents who have adopted them

Blended families include children who live with one biological or adoptive parent and a nonrelated stepparent who are married

Cohabitating families include children who live with one biological parent and a nonrelated adult who are cohabitating

Extended families include children living with one biological or adoptive parent and a related adult who is not their parent (grandparent, aunt, uncle)

Other families include children living with related or nonrelated adults who are neither biological nor adoptive parents (grandparents, adult siblings, foster parents) Family is the first system to which a person is attached and is the most influential system to which an individual will belong.

- Families go through various developmental stages. The roles the family members fulfill change throughout the stages. For instance, when adults become parents they care for and model behavior for their children. As children mature, they rely on their parents less. Later on, the parents may have to depend on their children to meet their needs.
- Families can have healthy or dysfunctional characteristics in one or more areas of functioning.
- Healthy family relationships support the well-being of each member of the family unit.

AREAS OF FUNCTIONING

Communication

HEALTHY FAMILIES: There are clear, understandable messages between family members, and each member is encouraged to express individual feelings and thoughts.

DYSFUNCTIONAL FAMILIES
One or more members use unhealthy patterns, including the following.
- **Blaming**: Members blame others to shift focus away from their own inadequacies.
- **Manipulating**: Members use dishonesty to support their own agendas.
- **Placating**: One member takes responsibility for problems to keep peace at all costs.
- **Distracting**: A member inserts irrelevant information during attempts at problem solving.
- **Generalizing**: Members use overall descriptions ("always" and "never") in describing family encounters.

Management

HEALTHY FAMILIES: Adults of a family agree on important issues (rule making, finances, plans for the future).

DYSFUNCTIONAL FAMILIES: Management can be chaotic, with a child making management decisions at times.

Boundaries

HEALTHY FAMILIES: Boundaries are distinguishable between family roles. Clear boundaries define roles of each member and are understood by all. Each family member is able to function appropriately.

DYSFUNCTIONAL FAMILIES
- **Enmeshed boundaries:** Thoughts, roles, and feelings blend so much that individual roles are unclear.
- **Rigid boundaries:** Rules and roles are completely inflexible. These families tend to have members who isolate themselves, and communication is minimal. Members do not share thoughts or feelings.

Socialization

HEALTHY FAMILIES: All members interact, plan, and adopt healthy ways of coping. Children learn to function as family members, as well as members of society. Members are able to change as the family grows and matures.

DYSFUNCTIONAL FAMILIES: Children do not learn healthy socialization skills within the family and have difficulty adapting to socialization roles of society.

Emotional/Supportive

HEALTHY FAMILIES: Emotional needs of family members are met most of the time, and members have concerns about each other. Conflict and anger do not dominate.

DYSFUNCTIONAL FAMILIES: Negative emotions predominate most of time. Members are isolated and afraid and do not show concern for each other.

OTHER CONCEPTS RELATED TO FAMILY DYSFUNCTION

Scapegoating: A member of the family with little power is blamed for problems within the family. For example, one child who has not completed their chores can be blamed for the entire family not being able to go on an outing.

Triangulation: A third party is drawn into the relationship with two members whose relationship is unstable. For example, one parent can develop an alliance with a child, leaving the other parent relatively uninvolved with both.

Multigenerational issues: These are emotional issues or themes within a family that continue for at least three generations (a pattern of substance use or addictive behavior, dysfunctional grief patterns, triangulation patterns, divorce).

DISCIPLINE

Disciplining children is a family behavior that can be healthy or dysfunctional. Setting limits on children's behavior protects their safety and provides them with security. Discipline should be consistent, timely, and age-appropriate. Parents should administer discipline in private, when they are calm. Caregivers should be in unison on when and how to discipline.

FAMILY THERAPY

A family is defined as a group with reciprocal relationships in which members are committed to each other. Examples of families vary widely and are often nontraditional (e.g., a family made up of a child living with a grown brother and his partner). Areas of functioning for families include management, boundaries, communication, emotional support, and socialization. Dysfunction can occur in any one or more areas.

- In family therapy, the focus is on the family as a system, rather than on each person as an individual.
- Family data collection includes focused interviews and use of various family assessment tools.
- Nurses work with families to provide teaching. For example, an RN might instruct a family on medication administration or ways to help a family member manage their mental health disorder. ⓠpcc
- Nurses also work to mobilize family resources, to improve communication, and to strengthen the family's ability to cope with the illness of one member.
- Multi-family therapy is an effective modality for families who are experiencing similar challenges. For example, two or more families learn new skills and share their experience of living with a family member who is diagnosed with a serious mental illness like schizophrenia.

Application Exercises

1. A nurse wants to use democratic leadership with a group whose purpose is to learn appropriate conflict resolution techniques. The nurse is correct in implementing this form of group leadership when demonstrating which of the following actions?

   A. Observes group techniques without interfering with the group process

   B. Discusses a technique and then directs members to practice the technique

   C. Asks for group suggestions of techniques and then supports discussion

   D. Suggests techniques and asks group members to reflect on their use

2. A nurse is assisting in planning group therapy for clients dealing with bereavement. Which of the following activities should the nurse include in the initial phase? (Select all that apply.)

   A. Encourage the group to work toward goals.

   B. Define the purpose of the group.

   C. Discuss termination of the group.

   D. Identify informal roles of members within the group.

   E. Establish an expectation of confidentiality within the group.

3. A nurse is working with an established group and identifies various member roles. Which of the following should the nurse identify as an individual role?

   A. A member who praises input from other members.

   B. A member who follows the direction of other members.

   C. A member who brags about accomplishments.

   D. A member who evaluates the group's performance toward a standard.

4. A nurse on an acute mental health unit forms a group to focus on self-management of medications. At each of the meetings, two of the members conspire together to exclude the rest of the group. This is an example of which of the following concepts?

   A. Triangulation

   B. Group process

   C. Subgroup

   D. Hidden agenda

5. A nurse is assisting with a family therapy session. The younger child tells the nurse about plans to make the older sibling look bad, believing this will earn more freedom and privileges. The nurse should identify this dysfunctional behavior as which of the following?

   A. Placation

   B. Manipulation

   C. Blaming

   D. Distraction

Active Learning Scenario

A nurse is contributing to the plan of care for a family that is planning to begin therapy to improve the emotional and supportive aspect of the family unit. Use the ATI Active Learning Template: Basic Concept to complete this item.

RELATED CONTENT: Identify the definition of a family.

UNDERLYING PRINCIPLES: Discuss the focus of family therapy.

NURSING INTERVENTIONS

- Identify at least two outcomes for emotional/supportive functioning.

- Identify at least two interventions to assist the family during therapy.

Active Learning Scenario Key

Using the ATI Active Learning Template: Basic Concept

RELATED CONTENT: A family is defined as a group with reciprocal relationships in which members are committed to each other.

UNDERLYING PRINCIPLES
- Family needs and problems within family dynamics
- Improve family functioning

NURSING INTERVENTIONS
- Outcomes
  - Family members will have emotional needs met the majority of the time.
  - Family members will show concern for each other.
  - Family members will maintain a positive emotional atmosphere rather than one of conflict and anger.
- Interventions
  - Instruct the family effective ways to deal with emotional needs of family members.
  - Assist the family to improve understanding among family members.
  - Promote positive interaction among family members.
  - Identify common feelings, experiences, and thoughts among family members.

Ⓝ *NCLEX® Connection: Psychosocial Integrity, Support Systems*

Application Exercises Key

1. C. **CORRECT:** When taking action to resolve conflict resolution techniques, the nurse should use democratic leadership supports group interaction and decision making to solve problems. Laissez-faire leadership allows the group process to progress without any attempt by the leader to control the direction of the group. Autocratic leadership controls the direction of the group.

   Ⓝ *NCLEX® Connection: Psychosocial Integrity, Behavioral Management*

2. B, C, E. **CORRECT:** During the initial phase the nurse should, identify the purpose of the group, set the tone of the group, including an expectation of confidentiality and discuss termination of the group. During the working phase, the group works toward goals, and identify informal roles that other members in the group often assume.

   Ⓝ *NCLEX® Connection: Psychosocial Integrity, Grief and Loss*

3. C. **CORRECT:** When evaluating functional roles of a group, the nurse should identify an individual who brags about accomplishments is acting in an individual role that does not promote the progression of the group toward meeting goals. An individual who praises the input of others is acting in a maintenance role. An individual who is a follower is acting in a maintenance role. An individual who evaluates the group's performance is acting in a task role.

   Ⓝ *NCLEX® Connection: Psychosocial Integrity, Behavioral Management*

4. C. **CORRECT:** A subgroup is a small number of people within a larger group who function separately from that group. Triangulation is when a third party is drawn into a relationship with two members whose relationship is unstable. Group process is the verbal and nonverbal communication that occurs within the group during group sessions. A hidden agenda is when some group members have a different goal than the stated group goals. The hidden agenda is often disruptive to the effective functioning of the group.

   Ⓝ *NCLEX® Connection: Psychosocial Integrity, Behavioral Management*

5. B. **CORRECT:** The nurse should identify, manipulation is the dysfunctional behavior of using dishonesty to support an individual agenda. Placation is the dysfunctional behavior of taking responsibility for problems to keep peace among family members. Blaming is the dysfunctional behavior of blaming others to shift focus away from the individual's own inadequacies. Distraction is the dysfunctional behavior of inserting irrelevant information during attempts at problem solving.

   Ⓝ *NCLEX® Connection: Psychosocial Integrity, Behavioral Management*

UNIT 2   TRADITIONAL NONPHARMACOLOGICAL
          THERAPIES

CHAPTER 9 *Stress Management*

Stress is the brain's natural response to any demand. Stressors are physical or psychological factors that produce stress. Any stressor, whether it is perceived as "good" or "bad," produces a biological response in the body. Individuals need the presence of some stressors to provide interest and purpose to life; however, too much stress or too many stressors can cause distress. Anxiety and anger are damaging stressors that cause distress.

The body responds to a perceived or actual threat by activating the fight-or-flight response. If stress is prolonged, maladaptive responses can occur.

Stress management is a client's ability to experience appropriate emotions and cope with stress. The client who manages stress in a healthy manner is flexible and uses a variety of coping techniques or mechanisms. Responses to stress and anxiety are affected by factors (age, gender, culture, life experiences, and lifestyle). The effects of stressors are cumulative. For example, the death of a family member can cause a high amount of stress. If the client experiencing that stress is also experiencing other stressful events at the same time, this could cause illness due to the cumulative effect of those stressors.

A client's ability to use successful stress management techniques can improve stress-related medical conditions and improve functioning. Viewing a stressor as positive appears to be the result of adaptation or learning, also known as preconditioning, from previous stressful experiences. For example, a short-term or acute stress response, such as preparing to make a speech or take an exam, allows a person to be at a high level of mental and physical performance.

DATA COLLECTION

Protective factors increasing a client's resilience, or ability to resist the effects of stress, include the following.
- Physical health
- Strong sense of self
- Religious or spiritual beliefs
- Optimism
- Hobbies and other outside interests
- Satisfying interpersonal relationships
- Strong social support systems
- Humor

An individual's response can be described as fight, faint, flight, freeze, or fawn.
- Fight: facing the stressor or situation ready to confront or fight
- Faint: limiting exposure to stress by physically fainting, or experiencing syncope
- Flight: running away from or fleeing the stressor or situation
- Freeze: unable to respond or react against the stressor or situation
- Fawn: attempting to please or give in to the stressor or situation

EXPECTED FINDINGS

ACUTE STRESS (FIGHT OR FLIGHT)
- Apprehension
- Unhappiness or sorrow
- Decreased appetite
- Increased respiratory rate, heart rate, cardiac output, blood pressure
- Increased metabolism and glucose use
- Depressed immune system

PROLONGED STRESS (MALADAPTIVE RESPONSE)
- Chronic anxiety or panic attacks
- Depression, chronic pain, sleep disturbances
- Weight gain or loss
- Increased risk for myocardial infarction, stroke
- Poor diabetes control, hypertension, fatigue, irritability, decreased ability to concentrate
- Chronic exposure to stress hormones, specifically cortisol, weakens the immune system, resulting in increased susceptibility to illness and infection

STANDARDIZED SCREENING TOOLS

Life-changing events questionnaires (the Holmes and Rahe stress scale) to measure Life Change Units, Perceived Stress Scale, and Lazarus's Cognitive Appraisal. The use of stress scales can provide the nurse with insight into their client's experience of stress and risk for developing an illness. It is a useful part of the client's plan of care for stress reduction and coping. Q(EBP)

PATIENT-CENTERED CARE

NURSING CARE

Most nursing care involves reinforcing teaching of stress-reduction strategies to clients.

Cognitive techniques

Cognitive reframing
- The client is helped to look at irrational cognitions (thoughts) in a more realistic light and to restructure those thoughts in a more positive way.
- As an example, a client can think they are "a terrible father to my daughter." A health professional, using therapeutic communication techniques, could help the client reframe that thought into a positive thought ("I've made some bad mistakes as a parent, but I've learned from them and have improved my parenting skills.").
- The nurse should encourage their client to learn to talk to themselves with kindness, rather than doubt or blame. Positive self-talk is linked to physical and mental health benefits.

Behavioral techniques

RELAXATION TECHNIQUES
- **Meditation** is a technique used to train the mind and help a greater calm. Meditation can help a client connect with their deep inner self and promote healing and strategies to cope with stress.
- **Guided imagery**: The client is guided through a series of images to promote relaxation. Images vary depending on the individual. For example, one client might imagine walking on a beach, while another client might imagine themselves in a position of success.
- **Breathing exercises** are used to decrease rapid breathing and promote relaxation.
- **Progressive muscle relaxation** is a technique used to achieve a relaxation response. This technique involves purposefully tensing specific muscle groups and then relaxing them in a progressive format. This can be performed with external feedback or without. Progressive muscle relaxation is an easy technique that can be performed almost anywhere.
- **Physical exercise** (yoga, walking, biking) causes release of endorphins that lower anxiety, promote relaxation, and have antidepressant effects.
- Use nursing judgment to determine the appropriateness of relaxation techniques for clients who are experiencing acute manifestations of a psychotic disorder. **Qs**

Journal writing
- Journaling has been shown to allow for a therapeutic release of stress. Journaling can ease anxiety, worry, and obsessional thinking. It also can increase confidence and hope.
- This activity can help the client identify stressors and make specific plans to decrease stressors.

Cognitive reframing
- The client learns to prioritize differently to reduce the number of stressors affecting them.
- For example, a person who is under stress due to feeling overworked might delegate some tasks to others rather than doing them all on their own.

Biofeedback

A nurse or other health professional trained in this method uses a sensitive mechanical device to assist the client to gain voluntary control of such autonomic functions as heart rate and blood pressure. Exercise gadgets and smart watches provide the ability to track sleep and heart rates.

Mindfulness
- The client is encouraged to be mindful of their surroundings using all of their senses (the relaxing warmth of sunlight or the sound of a breeze blowing through the trees).
- The client learns to restructure negative thoughts and interpretations into positive ones. For example, instead of saying, "It's so frustrating that the elevator isn't working," the client restructures the thought into, "Using the stairs is a great opportunity to burn off some extra calories."

Assertiveness training
- The client learns to communicate in a more assertive manner in order to decrease psychological stressors.
- For example, one technique teaches the client to assert their feelings by describing a situation or behavior that causes stress, discussing feelings about the behavior or situation, and then making a change. The client states, "When you keep telling me what to do, I feel angry and frustrated. I need to try making some of my own decisions."

Other individual stress-reduction techniques
- The nurse should assist each client in identifying individual strategies that improve the client's ability to cope with stress. **Qpcc**
- Examples include individual hobbies (fishing, scrapbooking), music therapy, pet therapy, sleep, massage, and aerobic exercise.

1. A nurse is assisting with an educational seminar on stress for other nursing staff. Which of the following information should the nurse recommend for inclusion?

    A. Excessive stressors cause the client to experience distress.

    B. The body's initial adaptive response to stress is denial.

    C. Absence of stressors results in homeostasis.

    D. Negative, rather than positive, stressors produce a biological response.

2. A nurse is discussing acute vs. prolonged stress with a client. Which of the following effects should the nurse identify as an acute stress response?

    A. Chronic pain

    B. Depressed immune system

    C. Increased blood pressure

    D. Panic attacks

    E. Unhappiness

3. A nurse is reinforcing teaching with a client about stress-reduction techniques. Which of the following client statements indicates understanding of the information?

    A. "Cognitive reframing will help me change my irrational thoughts to something positive."

    B. "Progressive muscle relaxation uses a mechanical device to help me gain control over my pulse rate."

    C. "Biofeedback causes my body to release endorphins so that I feel less stress and anxiety."

    D. "Mindfulness allows me to prioritize the stressors that I have in my life so that I have less anxiety."

4. A nurse is talking with a client who reports experiencing increased stress because a new partner is "pressuring me and my kids to go live with him. I love him, but I'm not ready to do that." Which of the following recommendations should the nurse make to promote a change in the client's situation?

    A. Learn to practice mindfulness.

    B. Use assertiveness techniques.

    C. Exercise regularly.

    D. Rely on the support of a close friend.

5. A nurse is caring for a client who states, "I'm so stressed at work because of my coworker. I am expected to finish others' work because of their laziness!" When discussing effective communication, which of the following statements by the client to the coworker indicates client understanding?

    A. "You really should complete your own work. I don't think it's right to expect me to complete your responsibilities."

    B. "Why do you expect me to finish your work? You must realize that I have my own responsibilities."

    C. "It is not fair to expect me to complete your work. If you continue, then I will report your behavior to our supervisor."

    D. "When I have to pick up extra work, I feel very overwhelmed. I need to focus on my own responsibilities."

Active Learning Scenario

A nurse is leading a peer group discussion about reinforcing teaching of stress-related strategies. Use the ATI Active Learning Template: Basic Concept to complete this item.

NURSING INTERVENTIONS: List 3 behavioral and relaxation techniques the nurse should recommend and how to explain their use to the client.

Active Learning Scenario Key

Using the ATI Active Learning Template: Basic Concept

NURSING INTERVENTIONS

- **Meditation** is a technique used to train the mind and help a greater calm. Meditation can help a client connect with their deep inner self and promote

- **Guided imagery:** The client is guided through a series of images to promote relaxation. Images vary depending on the individual. For example, one client might imagine walking on a beach, while another client might imagine themselves in a position of success.

- **Breathing exercises:** These are used to decrease rapid breathing and promote relaxation.

- **Progressive muscle relaxation:** This technique involves purposefully tensing specific muscle groups and then relaxing them in a progressive format. This can be performed with external feedback or without.

- **Physical exercise (yoga, walking, biking):** This causes the release of endorphins that lower anxiety, promote relaxation, and have antidepressant effects.

Use nursing judgment to determine the appropriateness of relaxation techniques for clients who are experiencing acute manifestations of a psychotic disorder.

Ⓝ *NCLEX® Connection: Psychosocial Integrity, Stress Management*

Application Exercises Key

1. A. **CORRECT:** When taking action and assisting with preparing an educational seminar on stress for other nursing staff, the nurse should discuss distress is the result of excessive or damaging stressors (anxiety or anger). Denial is part of the grief process. The body's initial adaptive response to stress is known as the fight-or-flight mechanism. Individuals need the presence of some stressors to provide interest and purpose to life. Both positive and negative stressors produce a biological response in the body.

   Ⓝ *NCLEX® Connection: Psychosocial Integrity, Stress Management*

2. B, C, E. **CORRECT:** When taking action and discussing acute vs. prolonged stress with a client, the nurse should identify an acute stress response as a depressed immune system, increased blood pressure, and unhappiness as indicators of acute stress. Chronic pain indicates a prolonged or maladaptive stress response. Panic attacks indicate a prolonged or maladaptive stress response.

   Ⓝ *NCLEX® Connection: Psychosocial Integrity, Stress Management*

3. A. **CORRECT:** When evaluating a client's understanding about stress reduction techniques, the nurse should identify that the client understands cognitive reframing helps the client look at irrational cognitions (thoughts) in a more realistic light and to restructure those thoughts in a more positive way. Biofeedback, rather than progressive muscle training, uses a mechanical device to promote voluntary control over autonomic functions. Physical exercise, rather than biofeedback, causes a release of endorphins that lower anxiety and reduce stress. Priority restructuring, rather than mindfulness, teaches the client to prioritize differently to reduce the number of stressors.

   Ⓝ *NCLEX® Connection: Psychosocial Integrity, Stress Management*

4. B. **CORRECT:** When taking actions and recommending means to promote change in a client's situation, the nurse should recommend to use assertive communication which allows the client to assert their feelings and then make a change in the situation. Mindfulness is appropriate to decrease the client's stress. However, it does not promote a change in the client's situation. Regular exercise is appropriate to decrease the client's stress. However, it does not promote a change in the client's situation. Social support is appropriate to decrease the client's stress. However, it does not promote a change in the client's situation.

   Ⓝ *NCLEX® Connection: Psychosocial Integrity, Stress Management*

5. D. **CORRECT:** When evaluating a client's understanding of effective communication, the nurse should identify the client indicates an understanding when the response demonstrates assertive communication, which allows the client to state their feelings about the behavior and then promote a change. Disapproving/disagreeing can prompt a defensive reaction and is therefore nontherapeutic. "Why" questions imply criticism and can prompt a defensive reaction and is therefore nontherapeutic. Aggressive and threatening responses can prompt a defensive reaction and is therefore nontherapeutic.

   Ⓝ *NCLEX® Connection: Psychosocial Integrity, Therapeutic Communication*

CHAPTER 10 ## Brain Stimulation Therapies

Brain stimulation therapies offer a nonpharmacological treatment for clients who have certain mental health disorders. Brain stimulation therapies include electroconvulsive therapy (ECT), repetitive transcranial magnetic stimulation (RTMS), vagus nerve stimulation (VNS), and deep brain stimulation (DBS).

Electroconvulsive therapy

ECT uses electrical current to induce brief seizure activity while the client is anesthetized. The exact mechanism of ECT is still unknown. One theory suggests that the seizure activity produced by ECT can enhance the effects of neurotransmitters (serotonin, dopamine, and norepinephrine) in the brain.

INDICATIONS

POTENTIAL DIAGNOSES

Major depressive disorder

- Clients whose manifestations are not responsive to pharmacological treatment
- Clients for whom the risks of other treatments outweigh the risks of ECT
- Clients who are suicidal or homicidal and for whom there is a need for rapid therapeutic response Q EBP
- Clients who are experiencing psychotic manifestations

Schizophrenia spectrum disorders

- Clients who have schizophrenia with catatonic manifestations
- Clients who have schizoaffective disorder

Acute manic episodes

- Clients who have bipolar disorder with rapid cycling (four or more episodes of acute mania within 1 year)
- Clients who are unresponsive to treatment with lithium and antipsychotic medications

CONTRAINDICATIONS

There are no absolute contraindications. However, the nurse should collect data regarding medical conditions that place clients at higher risk of adverse effects. These conditions include the following.
- **Cardiovascular disorders:** Recent myocardial infarction, hypertension, heart failure, cardiac arrhythmias. ECT increases the stress on the heart due to seizure activity that occurs during the treatment.
- **Cerebrovascular disorders:** History of stroke, brain tumor, subdural hematoma. ECT increases intracranial pressure and blood flow through the brain during treatment.

Mental health conditions for which ECT has not been found useful include the following.
- Substance use disorders
- Personality disorders
- Dysphoric disorder

CONSIDERATIONS

PROCEDURAL CARE

- The typical course of ECT treatment is two to three times a week for a total of 6 to 12 treatments for depression.
- The provider obtains informed consent. If ECT is involuntary, the provider can obtain consent from next of kin or a court order.
- Pre-ECT work up can include a chest x-ray, blood work, ECG. Benzodiazepines should be discontinued as they will interfere with the seizure process.
- **Medication management**
  - Thirty minutes prior to the beginning of the procedure, an IM injection of atropine sulfate or glycopyrrolate is administered to decrease secretions that could cause aspiration and to counteract any vagal stimulation effects (bradycardia). Q s
  - At the time of the procedure, an anesthesia provider administers a short-acting anesthetic (etomidate or propofol) via IV bolus.
  - A muscle relaxant (succinylcholine) is then administered to paralyze the client's muscles during the seizure activity, which decreases the risk for injury. Succinylcholine paralyzes the respiratory muscles so the client requires assistance with breathing and oxygenation.
- Severe hypertension should be controlled because a short period of hypertension occurs immediately after the ECT procedure.
- Any cardiac conditions (dysrhythmias or hypertension) should be monitored and treated before the procedure.
- The nurse monitors vital signs and mental status before and after the ECT procedure.

- The nurse collects data regarding the client's and family's understanding and knowledge of the procedure and provides reinforcement as necessary. Many clients and family have misconceptions about ECT due to media portrayals of the procedure. Due to the use of anesthesia and muscle relaxants, the tonic-clonic seizure activity associated with the procedure in the past is no longer an effect of the treatment.
- An IV line is inserted and maintained until full recovery.
- Electrodes are applied to the scalp for electroencephalogram (EEG) monitoring.
- The client receives 100% oxygen during and after ECT until the return of spontaneous respirations.
- Ongoing cardiac monitoring is provided, including blood pressure, electrocardiogram (ECG), and oxygen saturation.
- Clients are expected to become alert about 15 min following ECT.

COMPLICATIONS

Memory loss and confusion

Short-term memory loss, confusion, and disorientation occurs immediately following the procedure can persist for several hours. Clients have retrograde amnesia which is the loss of memory of events leading up to the procedure and have no memory of the procedure. Memory loss can persist for several weeks. Whether ECT causes permanent memory loss is controversial, but most clients fully recover from any memory deficits.

NURSING ACTIONS
- Provide frequent orientation.
- Provide a safe environment to prevent injury. Qs
- Assist the client with personal hygiene as needed.

Reactions to anesthesia

NURSING ACTIONS: Provide continuous monitoring during the procedure and in the immediate recovery phase.

Cardiovascular changes

NURSING ACTIONS: Monitor vital signs and cardiac rhythm regularly per protocol.

Relapse of depression

CLIENT EDUCATION: ECT is not a permanent cure. Weekly or monthly maintenance ECT can decrease the incidence of relapse.

Repetitive transcranial magnetic stimulation

RTMS is a noninvasive therapy that uses magnetic pulsations (MRI strength) to stimulate the cerebral cortex of the brain.

INDICATIONS

RTMS is approved by the United States Food and Drug Administration (FDA) for the treatment of major depressive disorder for clients who are not responsive to pharmacological treatment. TMS is similar to ECT but does not induce seizure activity.

CONSIDERATIONS

Reinforce teaching with the client about TMS.
- RTMS is commonly prescribed 3 to 5 days a week for a period of 4 to 6 weeks.
- RTMS can be performed as an outpatient procedure.
- The RTMS procedure lasts 30 to 40 min.
- A noninvasive electromagnet is placed on the client's scalp, allowing the magnetic pulsations to pass through.
- The client is alert during the procedure.
- Clients might feel a tapping or knocking sensation in the head, scalp skin contraction, and tightening of the jaw muscles during the procedure.
- RTMS, coupled with psychotherapy, has been shown to be very effective in treatment of depression.

COMPLICATIONS

- Common adverse effects include mild discomfort or a tingling sensation at the site of the electromagnet and headaches.
- Monitor for lightheadedness after the procedure.
- Seizures are a rare but potential complication.
- Clients with a history of seizure disorders should use low-frequency RTMS.
- RTMS is not associated with systemic adverse effects or neurologic deficits. RTMS is contraindicated for clients who have cochlear implants, brain stimulators, or medication pumps because the metal in the devices can interfere with the treatment.

Vagus nerve stimulation

- VNS provides electrical stimulation through the vagus nerve to the brain through a device that is surgically implanted under the skin on the client's chest similar to a pacemaker device.
- VNS is believed to result in an increased level of neurotransmitters and enhances the actions of antidepressant medications.

INDICATIONS

- Depression that is resistant to pharmacological treatment and/or ECT. The treatment is approved by the FDA.
- Current research studies are determining the effectiveness for VNS in clients who have anxiety disorders, obesity, and pain.

CONSIDERATIONS

Reinforce teaching with the client about VNS.
- VNS is commonly performed as an outpatient surgical procedure.
- The VNS device delivers around-the-clock programmed pulsations, usually every 5 min for a duration of 30 seconds.
- Therapeutic antidepressant effects usually take several weeks to achieve.
- The client can turn off the VNS device at any time by placing a special external magnet over the site of the implant.

COMPLICATIONS

- Voice changes due to the proximity of the implanted lead on the vagus nerve to the larynx and pharynx.
- Other potential adverse effects include hoarseness, throat or neck pain, and coughing. These commonly improve with time.
- Dyspnea, especially with physical exertion, is possible. Therefore, the client might want to turn off the VNS during exercise or when periods of prolonged speaking are required. Qs

Deep brain stimulation

- DBS is a treatment that surgically implants electrodes into the brain to stimulate underactive regions. These regions, which are underperforming in clients with depression, then function better. VNS is believed to result in an increased level of neurotransmitters and enhances the actions of antidepressant medications.
- This device is more invasive than the VNS and is implanted surgically, so it is reserved for clients who have tried many other treatments that have failed. The nurse should use standard postoperative care for these clients.

INDICATIONS

The treatment is approved by the FDA for Parkinson disease and treatment-resistant obsessive-compulsive disorder.

CONSIDERATIONS

- Educate the client about DBS.
  - DBS is commonly performed as an outpatient surgical procedure.
  - The DBS device delivers around-the-clock programmed pulsations, usually every 5 minutes for a duration of 30 seconds.
  - Therapeutic antidepressant effects usually take several weeks to achieve.
  - The client can turn off the DBS device at any time by placing a special external magnet over the site of the implant.
- Assist the provider in obtaining informed consent.

COMPLICATIONS

- The pulse generators that are installed pose a risk for infection.
- It is possible for the client to experience hypomania without a history of bipolar disorder.
- Other potential adverse effects include headaches, seizures, stroke, and confusion.

Active Learning Scenario

A nurse is preparing to assist in providing electroconvulsive therapy (ECT) treatment for a client. Use the ATI Active Learning Template: Therapeutic Procedure to complete this item.

DESCRIPTION OF PROCEDURE

NURSING INTERVENTIONS
- Identify two preprocedure medication management actions.
- Identify at least two intraprocedure actions.

Application Exercises

1. A nurse is reinforcing teaching to a client who is scheduled to receive ECT for the treatment of major depressive disorder. Which of the following client statements indicates understanding of the information provided?
   - A. "It is common to treat depression with ECT before trying medications."
   - B. "I can have my depression cured if I receive a series of ECT treatments."
   - C. "I should receive ECT once a week for 6 weeks."
   - D. "I will receive a muscle relaxant to protect me from injury during ECT."

2. A nurse is collecting data from a client following an ECT procedure. Which of the following findings should the nurse expect? (Select all that apply.)
   - A. Hypotension
   - B. Paralytic ileus
   - C. Memory loss
   - D. Polyuria
   - E. Confusion

3. A nurse is attending a peer group discussion about the indications for ECT. Which of the following indications should the nurse recommend for inclusion in the discussion?
   - A. Borderline personality disorder
   - B. Acute withdrawal related to a substance use disorder
   - C. Bipolar disorder with rapid cycling
   - D. Dysphoric disorder

4. A charge nurse is discussing RTMS with a newly licensed nurse. Which of the following statements by the newly licensed nurse indicates an understanding of the teaching?
   - A. "RTMS is indicated for clients who have schizophrenia spectrum disorders."
   - B. "I will provide postanesthesia care following RTMS."
   - C. "RTMS treatments usually last 5 to 10 minutes."
   - D. "I will schedule the client for RTMS treatments 3 to 5 times a week for the first several weeks."

5. A nurse is contributing to the plan of care for a client following surgical implantation of a VNS device. The nurse should plan to monitor for which of the following adverse effects? (Select all that apply.)
   - A. Voice changes
   - B. Seizure activity
   - C. Disorientation
   - D. Cough
   - E. Neck pain

Application Exercises Key

1. D. **CORRECT:** When evaluating a client's understanding of ECT, the following information indicates an understanding of the procedure by the client. A muscle relaxant (succinylcholine) is administered to reduce the risk for injury during induced seizure activity. ECT is indicated for clients who have major depressive disorder and who are not responsive to pharmacological treatment. ECT does not cure depression. However, it can reduce the incidence and severity of relapse. The typical course of ECT treatment is two to three times a week for a total of six to 12 treatments.

   Ⓝ *NCLEX® Connection: Reduction of Risk Potential, Potential for Complications of Diagnostic Tests/Treatments/Procedures*

2. C, E. **CORRECT:** When collecting data for a client immediately following ECT, the nurse should expect the following findings: Transient short-term memory loss is an expected finding immediately following ECT. Confusion is an expected finding immediately following ECT. Immediately following ECT, the client's blood pressure is expected to be elevated. Paralytic ileus is not an expected finding of ECT. Polyuria is not an expect finding of ECT.

   Ⓝ *NCLEX® Connection: Reduction of Risk Potential, Potential for Complications of Diagnostic Tests/Treatments/Procedures*

3. C. **CORRECT:** When taking action and discussing indications for ECT with a peer group, the nurse should include the following information: ECT is indicated for the treatment of bipolar disorder with rapid cycling. ECT has not been found to be effective for the treatment of personality disorders, the treatment of substance use disorders, or dysphoric disorder.

   Ⓝ *NCLEX® Connection: Psychosocial Integrity, Behavioral Management*

4. D. **CORRECT:** When evaluating a client's understanding for RTMS, the following information indications an understanding of the procedure by the client. RTMS is commonly prescribed 3 to 5 times a week for the first four to six weeks. RTMS is indicated for the treatment of major depressive disorder that is not responsive to pharmacological treatment. ECT is indicated for the treatment of schizophrenia spectrum disorders. Postanesthesia care is not necessary after RTMS because the client does not receive anesthesia and is alert during the procedure. The RTMS procedure lasts 30 to 40 min.

   Ⓝ *NCLEX® Connection: Reduction of Risk Potential, Therapeutic Procedures*

5. A, D, E. **CORRECT:** When planning care for a client following surgical implantation of a VNS device, the nurse should monitor for the following adverse effects which include: Voice changes are a common adverse effect of VNS due to the proximity of the implanted lead on the vagus nerve to the larynx and pharynx. Coughing and neck pain are potential adverse effect of VNS. However, neck pain usually subsides with time. Seizure activity is associated with ECT rather than VNS. Disorientation is associated with ECT rather than VNS.

   Ⓝ *NCLEX® Connection: Reduction of Risk Potential, Potential for Complications of Diagnostic Tests/Treatments/Procedures*

Active Learning Scenario Key

Using the ATI Active Learning Template: Therapeutic Procedure

DESCRIPTION OF PROCEDURE: ECT is a nonpharmacological brain stimulation therapy for the treatment of mental health disorders, especially major depressive disorder. ECT induces seizure activity, which is thought to enhance the effects of neurotransmitters in the brain.

NURSING INTERVENTIONS

- Preprocedure medication management actions
  - Inform the client that atropine sulfate or glycopyrrolate will be administered 30 min prior to ECT.
  - Ensure the client has IV access prior to ECT.
  - Inform the client that the anesthesia provider will administer a short-acting anesthetic (etomidate or propofol) via IV bolus.
  - Inform the client that a muscle relaxant (succinylcholine) is administered to paralyze the client's muscles during the seizure activity, which decreases the risk for injury.
- Intraprocedure actions
  - Apply electrodes to the scalp for EEG monitoring.
  - Apply cardiac electrodes for ECG monitoring.
  - Assist with the administration of 100% oxygen during and after ECT until the return of spontaneous respirations.
  - Monitor vital signs.

Ⓝ *NCLEX® Connection: Reduction of Risk Potential, Potential for Complications of Diagnostic Tests/Treatments/Procedures*

When reviewing the following chapters, keep in mind the relevant topics and tasks of the NCLEX outline.

Health Promotion and Maintenance

HEALTH PROMOTION/DISEASE PREVENTION: Identify risk factors for disease/illness.

SELF-CARE: Monitor client ability to perform instrumental activities of daily living.

COMMUNITY RESOURCES: Identify community resources for clients.

Psychosocial Integrity

BEHAVIORAL MANAGEMENT
Assist client in using behavioral strategies to decrease anxiety.

Assist client with achieving self–control of behavior.

CHEMICAL AND OTHER DEPENDENCIES/SUBSTANCE USE DISORDER
Identify signs and symptoms of substance abuse, chemical dependency, withdrawal, or toxicity.

Encourage client participation in support groups.

CRISIS INTERVENTION
Identify client in crisis.

Use crisis intervention techniques to assist client in coping.

MENTAL HEALTH CONCEPTS
Identify client symptoms of acute or chronic mental illness.

Assist in care of a client experiencing sensory/perceptual alterations.

Assist in the care of the cognitively impaired client.

THERAPEUTIC COMMUNICATION: Encourage client-appropriate use of verbal and nonverbal communication.

THERAPEUTIC ENVIRONMENT: Contribute to maintaining a safe and supportive environment for client.

ADVERSE EFFECTS/CONTRAINDICATIONS/SIDE EFFECTS/ INTERACTIONS: Monitor client for actual and potential adverse effects of medications.

EXPECTED ACTIONS/OUTCOMES: Reinforce education to client regarding medications.

UNIT 3   PSYCHOBIOLOGIC DISORDERS

CHAPTER 11 *Anxiety Disorders*

Normal anxiety is a healthy response to stress that is essential for survival. When anxiety is elevated or persistent, behavior changes and impairment of function can occur. These changes, known as anxiety disorders, tend to be persistent and often disabling.

Anxiety levels can be mild (restlessness, increased motivation, irritability), moderate (agitation, muscle tightness), severe (inability to function, ritualistic behavior, unresponsive), or panic (distorted perception, loss of rational thought, immobility).

TYPES OF DISORDERS

ANXIETY DISORDERS

Anxiety disorders recognized and defined by the DSM-5-TR include the following.
- **Separation anxiety disorder:** The client experiences excessive fear or anxiety when separated from an individual to whom the client is emotionally attached.
- **Specific phobias:** The client experiences an irrational fear of a certain object or situation. Specific clinical names are used to refer to specific phobias (monophobia = phobia of being alone; zoophobia = phobia of animals; acrophobia = phobia of heights).
- **Agoraphobia:** The client experiences extreme fear of at least 2 situations that is persistent and of which they feel escape is not possible or they may experience embarrassing incidents.
- **Social anxiety disorder:** The client experiences excessive fear of social or performance situations.
- **Panic disorder:** The client experiences recurrent panic attacks.
- **Generalized anxiety disorder (GAD):** The client exhibits uncontrollable, excessive worry for at least 6 months.

OBSESSIVE-COMPULSIVE DISORDERS

Obsessive-compulsive and related disorders are not actual anxiety disorders but have similar effects and include the following.
- **Obsessive-compulsive disorder (OCD):** The client has intrusive thoughts of unrealistic obsessions and tries to control these thoughts with compulsive behaviors, such as repetitive cleaning of a particular object or washing of hands.
- **Hoarding disorder:** The client has difficulty parting with possessions, resulting in extreme stress and functional impairments.
- **Body dysmorphic disorder:** The client has a preoccupation with perceived flaws or defects in physical appearance.

DATA COLLECTION

RISK FACTORS

- Most anxiety disorders are more likely to occur in females. Obsessive-compulsive and related disorders also affect females more than males with the exception of hoarding disorder, which has a higher prevalence rate among males. Anxiety and obsessive-compulsive disorders have a genetic and neurobiological link.
- Clients can experience anxiety due to an acute medical condition, (hyperthyroidism or pulmonary embolism). It is important to assess the manifestations of anxiety in a medical facility to rule out a physical cause. Q EBP
- Trauma or negative life experiences such as adverse childhood experiences
- Lifestyle choices including poor diet, exercise, and substance use
- Substance-induced anxiety is related to current use of a chemical substance or to withdrawal effects from a substance (alcohol).

EXPECTED FINDINGS

Separation anxiety disorder

- The client exhibits excessive levels of anxiety and concern when separated from someone to whom they have an emotional attachment, fearing that something tragic will occur resulting in permanent separation.
- The client's anxiety disrupts the ability to participate in routine daily activities.
- Physical manifestations of anxiety develop during the separation or in anticipation of the separation and include headaches, nausea and vomiting, and sleep disturbances.

Specific phobias

- The client reports a fear of specific objects (spiders, snakes, or strangers).
- The client reports a fear of specific experiences (flying, being in the dark, riding in an elevator, or being in an enclosed space).
- The client might experience anxiety manifestations just by thinking of the feared object or situation and might attempt to decrease the anxiety through the use of alcohol or other substances.

Agoraphobia

- The client avoids certain places or situations that cause anxiety. This avoidance might disrupt the client's ability to maintain employment or participate in routine activities of daily life.
- The client's fear and manifestations of anxiety are out of proportion with the actual danger of the place or situation.

Social anxiety disorder

- The client reports difficulty performing or speaking in front of others or participating in social situations due to an excessive fear of embarrassment or poor performance.
- The client might report physical manifestations (actual or factitious) in an attempt to avoid the social situation or need to perform.

Panic disorder

- Panic attacks typically last minutes but may occasionally continue for longer periods.
- Four or more of the following manifestations are present during a panic attack.
  ○ Palpitations
  ○ Shortness of breath
  ○ Choking or smothering sensation
  ○ Chest pain
  ○ Nausea
  ○ Feelings of depersonalization
  ○ Fear of dying or insanity
  ○ Chills or hot flashes
- The client might experience behavior changes and/or persistent worries about when the next attack will occur.

Generalized anxiety disorder

- The client exhibits uncontrollable, excessive worry for the majority of days over at least 6 months.
- GAD causes significant impairment in one or more areas of functioning (work-related duties).
- Manifestations of GAD include the following.
  ○ Restlessness
  ○ Muscle tension
  ○ Avoidance of stressful activities or events
  ○ Increased time and effort required to prepare for stressful activities or events
  ○ Procrastination in decision-making
  ○ Sleep disturbance

Obsessive-compulsive disorders

OCD: The client attempts to suppress persistent thoughts or urges that cause anxiety through compulsive or obsessive behaviors (repetitive handwashing). Obsessions or compulsions are time-consuming and result in impaired social and occupational functioning.

Hoarding disorder: The client has an obsessive desire to save items regardless of value and experiences extreme stress with thoughts of discarding or getting rid of items. The client's hoarding behavior results in social and occupational impairment and often leads to an unsafe living environment.

Body dysmorphic disorder: The client attempts to conceal a perceived physical flaw and practices repetitive behaviors (mirror checking or comparison to others) in response to the anxiety experienced over the perception. The client might have social and occupational impairment in response to the perceived physical defects or flaws.

STANDARDIZED SCREENING TOOLS

- Hamilton Rating Scale for Anxiety Q EBP
- Fear Questionnaire (phobias)
- Panic Disorder Severity Scale
- Yale-Brown Obsessive Compulsive Scale
- Hoarding Scale Self-Report

PATIENT-CENTERED CARE

NURSING CARE

- Providing trauma-informed care takes into consideration the client's experience and requires the nurse to be aware, sensitive, and responsive.
- Assist with conducting a structured interview to keep the client focused on the present.
- Collect data regarding a comorbid condition of substance use disorder.
- Provide safety and comfort to the client during the crisis period of these disorders, as clients in severe- to panic-level anxiety are unable to problem-solve and focus. Clients experiencing panic-level anxiety benefit from a calm, quiet environment.
- Remain with the client during the worst of the anxiety to provide reassurance.
- Determine the client's suicide risk. Qs
- Provide a safe environment for other clients and staff.
- Provide milieu therapy that employs the following.
  ○ Structured environment for physical safety and predictability
  ○ Monitoring for, and protection from, self-harm or suicide
  ○ Daily activities that encourage the client to share and be cooperative
  ○ Use of therapeutic communication skills (open-ended questions) to help the client express feelings of anxiety and to validate and acknowledge those feelings
  ○ Client participation in decision-making regarding care

- Use relaxation techniques with the client as needed for relief of pain, muscle tension, and feelings of anxiety.
- Instill hope for positive outcomes (but avoid false reassurance). Qpcc
- Enhance client self-esteem by encouraging positive statements and discussing past achievements.
- Assist the client to identify defense mechanisms that interfere with recovery.
- Postpone reinforcing health teaching until after acute anxiety subsides. Clients experiencing a panic attack or severe anxiety are unable to concentrate or learn.
- Identify counseling, group therapy, and other community resources for clients who have anxiety.

THERAPEUTIC PROCEDURES

Cognitive behavioral therapy

The anxiety response can be decreased by changing cognitive distortions. This therapy uses cognitive reframing to help the client identify negative thoughts that produce anxiety, examine the cause, and develop supportive ideas that replace negative self-talk. Qebp

Behavioral therapies

Behavioral therapies teach clients ways to decrease anxiety or avoidant behavior and allow an opportunity to practice techniques.
- **Relaxation training** is used to control pain, tension, and anxiety. Refer to the chapter on STRESS MANAGEMENT, which covers relaxation training techniques.
- **Modeling** allows a client to see a demonstration of appropriate behavior in a stressful situation. The goal of therapy is that the client will imitate the behavior.
- **Systematic desensitization** begins with mastering of relaxation techniques. Then, a client is exposed to increasing levels of an anxiety-producing stimulus (either imagined or real) and uses relaxation to overcome the resulting anxiety. The goal of therapy is that the client is able to tolerate a greater and greater level of the stimulus until anxiety no longer interferes with functioning. This form of therapy is especially effective for clients who have phobias.
- **Flooding** involves exposing the client to a great deal of an undesirable stimulus in an attempt to turn off the anxiety response. This therapy is useful for clients who have phobias.
- **Response prevention** focuses on preventing the client from performing a compulsive behavior with the intent that anxiety will diminish.
- **Thought stopping** teaches a client to say "stop" when negative thoughts or compulsive behaviors arise, and substitute a positive thought. The goal of therapy is that with time, the client uses the command silently.

CLIENT EDUCATION

- Monitor for manifestations of anxiety.
- Lifestyle management: helping the client make better choices, including nutritional strategies (healthy diet), exercise, and avoidance of excessive caffeine or substance use
- Defense mechanisms and coping strategies the client currently uses and strategies for better management of their anxiety
- Notify the provider of worsening effects and do not adjust medication dosages. Avoid stopping or increasing medication without consulting the provider.
- Assist the client to evaluate coping mechanisms that work and do not work for controlling the anxiety and learn new methods. Use of alternative stress relief and coping mechanisms might increase medication effectiveness and decrease the need for medication in most cases. Qpcc

Psychopharmacological Therapies

MAJOR MEDICATIONS TO TREAT ANXIETY DISORDERS

BENZODIAZEPINE SEDATIVE HYPNOTIC ANXIOLYTICS: Lorazepam, alprazolam, clonazepam, diazepam

ATYPICAL ANXIOLYTIC/NONBARBITURATE ANXIOLYTICS: Buspirone

SELECTED ANTIDEPRESSANTS
- **Selective serotonin reuptake inhibitors (SSRIs):** Paroxetine, sertraline, fluoxetine, citalopram, escitalopram, fluvoxamine
  ○ The first line of treatment for anxiety and obsessive-compulsive disorders
- **Serotonin norepinephrine reuptake inhibitors (SNRIs):** Venlafaxine, duloxetine, desvenlafaxine

OTHER CLASSIFICATIONS THAT MAY BE USED
- **Other antidepressants**
  ○ Tricyclic antidepressants (TCAs): Amitriptyline, imipramine, clomipramine
  ○ Monoamine oxidase inhibitors (MAOIs): Phenelzine
  ○ Antihistamines: Hydroxyzine pamoate, hydroxyzine hydrochloride
  ○ Mirtazapine
  ○ Trazodone
- **Beta blockers:** Propranolol
- **Peripherally acting antiadrenergics:** Prazosin
- **Anticonvulsants:** Gabapentin, pregabalin

Benzodiazepine sedative hypnotic anxiolytics

SELECT PROTOTYPE MEDICATION: Alprazolam

OTHER MEDICATIONS
- Diazepam
- Lorazepam
- Chlordiazepoxide
- Clorazepate
- Oxazepam
- Clonazepam

PURPOSE

EXPECTED PHARMACOLOGICAL ACTION:
Benzodiazepines enhance the inhibitory effects of gamma-aminobutyric acid in the central nervous system. Relief from anxiety occurs rapidly following administration.

THERAPEUTIC USES: Short-term treatment for generalized anxiety disorder and panic disorder

OTHER USES
- Seizure disorders
- Insomnia
- Muscle spasm
- Alcohol withdrawal (for prevention and treatment of acute manifestations)
- Induction of anesthesia
- Amnesic prior to surgery or procedures

COMPLICATIONS Qs

Central nervous system (CNS) depression

(Sedation, lightheadedness, ataxia, and decreased cognitive function)

CLIENT EDUCATION
- Observe for manifestations. Notify the provider if effects occur.
- Avoid hazardous activities (driving, operating heavy equipment/machinery).
- Avoid concurrent use of alcohol and other CNS depressants.
- Some formulas with a long-half life, like diazepam, may cause next-day sedation.

Anterograde amnesia

Difficulty recalling events that occur after dosing

CLIENT EDUCATION: Observe for manifestations. Notify the provider and withhold the medication if effects occur.

Acute toxicity

Oral toxicity: drowsiness, lethargy, confusion

IV toxicity: respiratory depression, severe hypotension, cardiac arrest.
- Benzodiazepines for IV use include diazepam and lorazepam.

NURSING ACTIONS
- For oral toxicity, gastric lavage is used, followed by the administration of activated charcoal or saline cathartics.
- Flumazenil is administered to counteract sedation and reverse the adverse effects.
- Monitor vital signs, maintain patent airway, and provide fluids to maintain blood pressure.
- Ensure availability of resuscitation equipment.

CLIENT EDUCATION: Watch for manifestations of toxicity. Notify the provider if these occur.

Paradoxical response

Insomnia, excitation, euphoria, anxiety, rage

CLIENT EDUCATION: Observe for indications. Notify the provider if paradoxical response occurs.

Withdrawal effects

- Anxiety, insomnia, diaphoresis, tremors, and lightheadedness, delirium and seizures
- Occurs infrequently with short-term use

CLIENT EDUCATION: After taking benzodiazepines regularly and in high doses, taper the dose over several weeks using a prescribed tapered dosing schedule.

CONTRAINDICATIONS/PRECAUTIONS

- Benzodiazepines are teratogenic medications because they can cause fetal risk. Because they are transmitted through human milk, they should not be taken by clients who are breastfeeding.
- Benzodiazepines are classified under Schedule IV of the Controlled Substances Act.
- Benzodiazepines are contraindicated in clients who have sleep apnea, respiratory depression, and/or glaucoma. Qs
- Use benzodiazepines cautiously in clients who have liver disease or a history of a substance use disorder.
- Benzodiazepines are generally used short-term due to the risk for dependence.
- Monitor fall risk for older adults who are prescribed benzodiazepines. Ⓖ

INTERACTIONS

CNS depressants (alcohol, barbiturates, opioids) can cause respiratory depression.

NURSING ACTIONS
- Avoid alcohol and other substances that cause CNS depression.
- Avoid hazardous activities (driving, operating heavy equipment/machinery).

NURSING ADMINISTRATION

- When discontinuing benzodiazepines that have been taken regularly for long periods and in higher doses, taper the dose over several weeks using a prescribed dosing schedule.
- Administer the medication with meals or snacks if GI upset occurs.

CLIENT EDUCATION
- Take the medication as prescribed and to avoid abrupt discontinuation of treatment to prevent withdrawal manifestations. Do not change the dosage or frequency without approval of the prescriber.
- Swallow sustained-release tablets and avoid chewing or crushing the tablets.
- Keep benzodiazepines in a secure place due to potential for misuse.
- Dependency can develop during and after treatment. Notify the provider if indications of withdrawal occur. Qs

Atypical anxiolytic/ nonbarbiturate anxiolytics

SELECT PROTOTYPE MEDICATION: Buspirone
- Buspirone is effective in managing anxiety and can be taken for long-term treatment of anxiety.

PURPOSE

EXPECTED PHARMACOLOGICAL ACTION
- The exact antianxiety mechanism is unknown. This medication binds to serotonin and dopamine receptors. There is less potential for dependency than with other anxiolytics. Use of buspirone does not result in sedation or potentiate the effects of other CNS depressants. It carries no risk of misuse.
- Antianxiety effects develop slowly. Initial responses take 1 week, and full effects take up to 4 weeks. As a result of this pharmacological action, buspirone needs to be taken on a scheduled basis and is not suitable for PRN usage.

THERAPEUTIC USES: Generalized anxiety disorder

COMPLICATIONS

CNS effects

Dizziness, nausea, headache, lightheadedness, agitation

NURSING ACTIONS: This medication does not interfere with activities because it does not cause sedation.

CONTRAINDICATIONS/PRECAUTIONS

- Buspirone is a teratogenic medication.
- Buspirone is not recommended for use by clients who are breastfeeding. Qs
- Use buspirone cautiously in clients who have liver or kidney dysfunction, as well as clients who have liver or renal dysfunction.
- Buspirone is contraindicated for concurrent use with MAOI antidepressants, or for 14 days after MAOIs are discontinued. Hypertensive crisis can result.

INTERACTIONS

Erythromycin, ketoconazole, St. John's wort, and grapefruit juice can increase the effects of buspirone.
- CLIENT EDUCATION
  - Avoid the use of erythromycin and ketoconazole.
  - Avoid herbal preparations containing St. John's wort.
  - Avoid drinking grapefruit juice.

NURSING ADMINISTRATION

Medication should be administered at the same time every day.

CLIENT EDUCATION
- Take the medication with meals to prevent gastric irritation.
- Effects do not occur immediately. It can take 1 week to notice first therapeutic effects, and up to 4 weeks to reach full therapeutic benefit. Medication should be taken on a regular basis, rather than an as-needed basis.
- Tolerance, dependence, or withdrawal manifestations are not an issue with this medication.

Active Learning Scenario

A nurse working in a mental health clinic is working with a client who experiences high levels of anxiety when riding in an elevator. What should the nurse reinforce with the client about the use of systematic desensitization as a form of behavioral therapy? Use the ATI Active Learning Template: Therapeutic Procedure to complete this item.

DESCRIPTION OF PROCEDURE

INDICATIONS: Describe one.

OUTCOMES/EVALUATION: Identify at least two client outcomes.

Application Exercises

1. A nurse observes a client who has OCD repeatedly applying, removing, and then reapplying makeup. The nurse identifies that repetitive behavior in a client who has OCD is due to which of the following underlying reasons?
   - A. Narcissistic behavior
   - B. Fear of rejection from staff
   - C. Attempt to reduce anxiety
   - D. Adverse effect of antidepressant medication

2. A nurse is collecting data for a client who has generalized anxiety disorder. Which of the following findings should the nurse expect? (Select all that apply.)
   - A. Excessive worry for 6 months
   - B. Impulsive decision-making
   - C. Delayed reflexes
   - D. Restlessness
   - E. Sleep disturbance

3. A nurse is caring for a client who is experiencing a panic attack. Which of the following actions should the nurse take?
   - A. Discuss new relaxation techniques.
   - B. Show the client how to change the behavior.
   - C. Distract the client with a television show.
   - D. Stay with the client and remain quiet.

4. A nurse is assisting in planning care for a client who has body dysmorphic disorder. Which of the following actions should the nurse plan to take first?
   - A. Collect data about the client's risk for self-harm.
   - B. Instill hope for positive outcomes.
   - C. Encourage the client to participate in group therapy sessions.
   - D. Assist the client to participate in treatment decisions.

5. A nurse is caring for a client who is to begin taking fluoxetine for treatment of panic disorders. Which of the following statements indicates the client understands the use of this medication?
   - A. "I will take the medication at bedtime."
   - B. "I will follow a low-sodium diet while taking this medication."
   - C. "I will need to discontinue this medication slowly."
   - D. "I will be at risk for weight loss with long-term use of this medication."

Application Exercises Key

1. C. **CORRECT:** When evaluating data, the nurse identifies that a client who has OCD repeats behaviors in an attempt to suppress persistent thoughts or urges that cause anxiety. Narcissism causes clients to seek admiration from others. Fear of rejection might cause a client to avoid social situations and might be associated with social phobia anxiety disorder. Clients who have OCD might take an antidepressant to help control repetitive behavior.

   Ⓝ *NCLEX® Connection: Psychosocial Integrity, Mental Health Concepts*

2. A, D, E. **CORRECT:** When collecting data for a client who has generalized anxiety disorder, the nurse should expect the following findings: uncontrollable, excessive worry for more than 6 months; restlessness; muscle tension; procrastination in decision-making; and the presence of sleep disturbances (the inability to fall asleep).

   Ⓝ *NCLEX® Connection: Psychosocial Integrity, Mental Health Concepts*

3. D. **CORRECT:** When taking action and caring for the client who is experiencing a panic attack, the nurse should quietly remain with the client. This promotes safety and reassurance without additional stimuli. The client is unable to concentrate on learning new information. Avoid further stimuli that can increase the client's level of anxiety.

   Ⓝ *NCLEX® Nursing Connection: Psychosocial Integrity, Behavioral Management*

4. A. **CORRECT:** The greatest risk to a client who has an anxiety or obsessive-compulsive disorder is self-harm or suicide. Therefore, the first action to take is to assess the client's risk for self-harm to ensure that the client is provided with a safe environment. Instill hope for positive outcomes, without providing false reassurance, as part of milieu therapy; however, there is another action to take first. Encourage the client to participate in group therapy to assist the client in order to address social impairments that result from the disorder; however, there is another action to take first. Encourage the client to participate in treatment decisions as part of milieu therapy; however, there is another action to take first.

   Ⓝ *NCLEX® Connection: Psychosocial Integrity, Mental Health Concepts*

5. C. **CORRECT:** When discontinuing fluoxetine, the client should taper the medication slowly according to a prescribed tapered dosing schedule to reduce the risk of withdrawal syndrome. The client should take fluoxetine in the morning to minimize sleep disturbances. The client is at risk for hyponatremia while taking fluoxetine. The client is at risk for weight gain, rather than loss, with long-term use of fluoxetine.

   Ⓝ *NCLEX® Connection: Pharmacological Therapies, Expected Actions/Outcomes*

Active Learning Scenario Key

Using the ATI Active Learning Template: Therapeutic Procedure

DESCRIPTION OF PROCEDURE: Systematic desensitization is a behavioral therapy that exposes clients to increasing levels of an anxiety-producing stimulus.

INDICATIONS: Systematic desensitization is indicated for the treatment of anxiety disorders associated with an anxiety-producing stimulus (a specific phobia).

OUTCOMES/EVALUATION
- The client will demonstrate effective relaxation techniques to overcome anxiety.
- The client's level of functioning will not be impaired by the phobia.
- The client will verbalize decreased feelings of anxiety when encountering the stimulus.

Ⓝ *NCLEX® Connection: Psychosocial Integrity, Stress Management*

UNIT 3   PSYCHOBIOLOGIC DISORDERS

CHAPTER 12 *Trauma- and Stressor-Related Disorders*

Clients can develop a trauma- or stressor-related disorder following exposure to an extreme stressor (perceived life-threatening events or interpersonal violence). In the setting of repeated exposure to toxic stress from adverse childhood experiences (ACEs), the brain undergoes changes that influence developing structures, altering health and behavior. It is important that nurses have an understanding of how to effectively assess and care for clients experiencing this type of disorder.

SPECIFIC DISORDERS

Acute stress disorder (ASD): Exposure to traumatic events causes anxiety, detachment and other manifestations about the event for at least 3 days but for not more than 1 month following the event.

Posttraumatic stress disorder (PTSD): Exposure to traumatic events causes anxiety, detachment, and other manifestations about the event for longer than 1 month following the event. Manifestations can last for years.

Adjustment disorder: A stressor triggers a reaction causing changes in mood and/or dysfunction in performing usual activities. The stressor and effects are less severe than with ASD or PTSD.

Dissociative disorders
- **Depersonalization/derealization disorder:** This disorder is characterized by a temporary change in awareness displaying depersonalization, derealization, or both, often in response to stress. Depersonalization is the feeling that a person is observing one's own personality or body from a distance. Derealization is the feeling that outside events are unreal or part of a dream, or that objects appear larger or smaller than they should.
- **Dissociative amnesia:** Inability to recall personal information related to traumatic or stressful events. The amnesia can be of events of a certain period of time or just certain details.
- **Dissociative fugue:** A type of dissociative amnesia in which the client travels to a new area and is unable to remember one's own identity and at least some of one's past. Can last weeks to months and usually follows a traumatic event
- **Dissociative identity disorder:** Client displays more than one distinct personality, with a stressful event precipitating the change from one personality to another.

Pediatric disorders
- **Reactive attachment disorder (RAD):** The child does not turn to an attachment figure (parent) for comfort or social interaction. Typically results in a child becoming withdrawn from adults or other caregivers due to unmet needs. Diagnosed before age 5: early childhood or infancy after 9 months of age
- **Disinhibited social engagement disorder (DSED):** Displays overly familiar behaviors toward strangers (or those relatively unfamiliar to them) without regard for appropriate social boundaries. Results from inadequate caregiving during childhood. Diagnosed during childhood after 9 months of age

HEALTH PROMOTION AND DISEASE PREVENTION

The nurse should monitor for and recognize child physical and sexual abuse, which can lead to ASD or PTSD, and report suspected cases to the proper authorities promptly to prevent severe trauma reactions from occurring.

The nurse should recognize occupations that have a high incidence of PTSD (military or first responders). Clients should receive support and treatment before severe trauma reactions occur.

PTSD PREVENTION

Health promotion measures to prevent PTSD during and after a traumatic incident (a mass casualty incident) Q EBP
- During the incident, be aware of need for breaks, rest, adequate water, and nutrition.
- Provide emotional support for those involved in the incident.
- Encourage staff to support each other.
- Debrief with others following the incident.
- Encourage expression of feelings by all involved.
- Use offered counseling resources.

DATA COLLECTION

RISK FACTORS

Adverse childhood experiences (ACEs) can result in psychological and behavioral manifestations in children, further creating stigma and creating a barrier that keeps children from accessing safe, stable, and supportive relationships. Those with the greatest risk for developing trauma-related disorders are women who have experienced four or more ACEs or have a history of interpersonal violence. ACEs have become a significant risk factor for the development of trauma-related disorders.

ASD, PTSD, and adjustment disorder

- Exposure to a traumatic event or experience (motor vehicle crash, sexual assault, physical abuse). For adjustment disorder, the event or experience can be less severe (breakup of a relationship or loss of employment).
- Exposure to trauma experienced during a natural disaster (fire, storm), or a man-made experience (terrorism).
- Exposure or repeated re-exposure to trauma in an occupational setting (experienced by medical personnel or law enforcement officers) can precipitate a trauma- and stressor-related disorder.
- Living through a traumatic event experienced by a family member or close friend (an airplane crash or homicide)
- PTSD is a risk factor for other disorders, including dissociative disorders, anxiety, depression, and substance use disorders.

ASD and PTSD

- Severity of the trauma (duration of the experience, the amount of personal threat associated with the trauma and whether it occurs far from home or in familiar surroundings)
- Individual vulnerabilities (past coping mechanisms, personality, and preexisting mental disorders)
- Insufficient treatment following the trauma (client social supports, societal attitudes about the situation, and cultural influences)

Adjustment disorder

- Pattern of life-long difficulty accepting change
- Learned pattern of difficulty with social skills or coping strategies, which, when a stressor occurs, can trigger a stress response out of proportion to the stressor

Dissociative disorders

- Traumatic life event
- Childhood abuse or trauma

EXPECTED FINDINGS

ASD and PTSD

- Intrusive findings (presence of memories, flashbacks, dreams about the traumatic event)
- Memories of the event recur involuntarily and are distressing to the client.
- Flashbacks (dissociative reactions where the client feels the traumatic event is recurring in the present), such as a military veteran feeling that they are reliving a combat situation after hearing a harmless loud noise
- Nighttime dreams related to the traumatic event
- Avoidance of people, places, events, or situations that bring back reminders of the traumatic event
- Trying to avoid thinking of the event

MOOD AND COGNITIVE ALTERATIONS

- Anxiety or depressive disorders
- Anger, irritability frequently present
- Decreased interest in current activities
- Guilt, negative self-beliefs, and cognitive distortions, such as "I am responsible for everything bad that happens."
- Detachment from others, including friends and family members
- Inability to experience positive emotional experiences, such as love and tenderness
- Dissociative manifestations (amnesia, derealization, depersonalization)

BEHAVIORAL MANIFESTATIONS

- Aggression, irritability, and angry responses toward others
- Hypervigilance with heightened startle responses
- Inability to focus and concentrate on work or other activities
- Sleep disturbances, such as insomnia
- Destructive behavior, such as suicidal thoughts or thoughts of harming others Qs

Adjustment disorder

- Depression
- Anxiety
- Changes in behavior (arguing with others or driving erratically)

Dissociative disorders

Depersonalization/derealization disorder: Reports of feeling detached from one's own body or of feeling that one's personal environment is unreal

Dissociative amnesia: Lack of memory that can range from name or date of birth to the client's entire lifetime

Dissociative identity disorder: Client displays two or more separate personalities. Each personality can be very distinct and different from the other

DIAGNOSTIC PROCEDURES

ASD, PTSD, and adjustment disorder QEBP

- Screening tools (the Primary Care PTSD Screen and the PTSD Checklist)
- Screening tests for anxiety and depression
- Asking about suicidal ideation
- Mental status examination

Dissociative disorders

- Physical data collection, electroencephalogram, and x-ray studies to rule out physical trauma (traumatic brain injury, epilepsy)
- Screening to rule out substance use
- Mental status examination and nursing history

NURSING ACTIONS

- Collect data about recent and remote memory for gaps or contradictions.
- Check for family and occupational difficulties.
- Ask about occurrence of stressful events.
- Monitor for depression, mood shifts, and anxiety.
- Use screening tools (the Cambridge Depersonalization Scale, Somatoform Dissociation Questionnaire, and the Dissociative Experiences Scale).

PATIENT-CENTERED CARE

NURSING CARE

Trauma-informed care involves care management that regards the impact of trauma for the client and addresses emotional, psychological, and physiological needs.

Universal trauma precautions

- Acknowledge and assume everyone has experienced trauma.
- Consider the tone of voice, eye contact, and body language in all communications.
- Respect culture, gender, race, ethnicity, and sexual orientation.
- Support client choices when possible.
- Minimize noise levels.
- Practice self-care and reach out to others when needed.

ASD, PTSD, and adjustment disorder Q̶EBP

- Establish a therapeutic relationship, and encourage the client to share feelings. Q̶PCC
- Provide a safe, nonthreatening, routine environment.
- Monitor clients for suicidal ideation, and take precautions as needed.
- Use multiple strategies to decrease anxiety (music therapy, guided imagery, massage, relaxation therapy, breathing techniques).
- If the client is a child, involve caregivers in treatment if possible, and use play, art, and other age-appropriate strategies to decrease stress.

Dissociative disorders

- During dissociative periods, assist the client with making decisions to lower stress.
- When the client shows readiness, encourage independence and decision-making.
- Assist with using grounding techniques (having the client clap hands or touch an object).
- Avoid giving the client too much information about past events to prevent increased stress. Q̶PCC

CLIENT EDUCATION

- Practice strategies to reduce anxiety.
- Verbalize negative feelings, and progress at own pace.

THERAPEUTIC PROCEDURES

Cognitive-behavioral therapy (cognitive restructuring): The client is helped to change distorted appraisal of events and negative thoughts.

Prolonged exposure therapy: Combines the use of relaxation techniques with exposure to the traumatic situation. The exposure can either be imagined through the use of repeated discussion of the traumatic event or practiced in real-world situations (in vivo) in which the client is exposed to the traumatic situation within safe limits. The repeated exposure eventually results in a decreased anxiety response.

Psychodynamic psychotherapy: Getting in touch with conscious and unconscious thought processes

Eye movement desensitization and reprocessing (EMDR)
- A therapy for both children and adults that uses rapid eye movements during desensitization techniques in a multi-phase process by a trained therapist
- Contraindicated for clients who have active suicidal ideation, psychosis, severe dissociative disorders, detached retina or glaucoma, or unstable substance use disorder Q̶EBP
- After developing a treatment plan, reinforce relaxation techniques to enhance client coping during next stages of EMDR.

Group or family therapy can include support groups or formal therapy.

Crisis intervention immediately following a traumatic incident

Somatic therapy for dissociative disorders: Psychotherapy works over time to increase awareness of the present and decrease dissociation episodes.

Hypnotherapy can be used for dissociative disorders.

Biofeedback/neurofeedback helps the client learn how to increase awareness and gain control of reactions to a trigger.

INTERPROFESSIONAL CARE

- Assist with referring clients to social workers/case managers for coordination of community care.
- Collaborate with psychotherapists to ensure coordination of care.

CLIENT EDUCATION

- Utilize relaxation techniques and other anxiety-reducing strategies.
- Monitor for causes and manifestations of the disorder.
- Avoid caffeine and alcohol.
- Perform grounding techniques for dissociative disorders. Observe and experience physical objects (touch a piece of ice, take a shower) or situations and keep a written journal to identify emotions associated with experiences.

MAJOR MEDICATIONS TO TREAT TRAUMA- AND STRESSOR-RELATED DISORDERS

ANTIDEPRESSANTS
- **Selective serotonin reuptake inhibitors:** Paroxetine, sertraline, fluoxetine, escitalopram, fluvoxamine
- **Serotonin norepinephrine reuptake inhibitor:** Venlafaxine
- **Tricyclic antidepressants:** Amitriptyline, imipramine
- **Monoamine oxidase inhibitor:** Phenelzine
- Noradrenergic and specific serotonergic antidepressant (NaSSA): Mirtazapine

BETA BLOCKERS: Propranolol, decreases elevated vital signs and manifestations of anxiety, panic, hypervigilance, and insomnia

PERIPHERALLY ACTING ANTIADRENERGICS: Prazosin, can decrease manifestations of hypervigilance and insomnia

CENTRALLY ACTING ADRENERGICS: Clonidine

Adjustment disorder and dissociative disorders

Medications might not be prescribed for adjustment disorder or the dissociative disorders unless specific findings of depression or anxiety require treatment.

Application Exercises

1. A nurse is assisting with a serious and prolonged mass casualty incident in the emergency department. Which of the following strategies should the nurse use to help prevent developing a trauma-related disorder? (Select all that apply.)
   A. Avoid thinking about the incident when it is over.
   B. Take breaks during the incident for food and water.
   C. Debrief with others following the incident.
   D. Avoid displays of emotion in the days following the incident.
   E. Take advantage of offered counseling.

2. A nurse working on an acute mental health unit is caring for a client who has posttraumatic stress disorder (PTSD). Which of the following findings should the nurse expect? (Select all that apply.)
   A. Difficulty concentrating on tasks
   B. Obsessive need to talk about the traumatic event
   C. Negative self-image
   D. Recurring nightmares
   E. Diminished reflexes

3. A nurse is assisting with collecting an admission history for a client who has acute stress disorder (ASD). Which of the following client behaviors should the nurse expect?
   A. The client remembers many details about the traumatic incident.
   B. The client expresses heightened elation about what is happening.
   C. The client remembers first noticing manifestations of the disorder 6 weeks after the traumatic incident occurred.
   D. The client expresses a sense of unreality about the traumatic incident.

4. A nurse is caring for a client who has derealization disorder. Which of the following findings should the nurse identify as an indication of derealization?
   A. The client describes a feeling of floating above the ground.
   B. The client has suspicions of being targeted in order to be killed and robbed.
   C. The client states that the furniture in the room seems to be small and far away.
   D. The client cannot recall anything that happened during the past 2 weeks.

5. A nurse in an acute mental health facility is planning care for a client who has dissociative fugue. Which of the following interventions should the nurse add to the plan of care?
   A. Reinforce teaching the client to recognize how stress brings on a personality change in the client.
   B. Repeatedly present the client with information about past events.
   C. Make decisions for the client regarding routine daily activities.
   D. Work with the client on grounding techniques.

6. A nurse is caring for a client who takes paroxetine to treat posttraumatic stress disorder. The client states, "I grind my teeth during the night, which causes pain in my mouth." The nurse should identify which of the following interventions as possible measures to manage the client's bruxism? (Select all that apply.)
   A. Concurrent administration of buspirone
   B. Administration of a different SSRI
   C. Use of a mouth guard
   D. Changing to a different class of antianxiety medication
   E. Increasing the dose of paroxetine

Application Exercises Key

1. **B, C, E. CORRECT:** Taking breaks and remembering to drink water and eat nutritious foods while working during a traumatic incident can help prevent development of a trauma-related disorder. Debriefing with others following a traumatic incident can help prevent development of a trauma-related disorder. Taking advantage of counseling offered by an employer or others can help prevent development of a trauma-related disorder. Thinking and talking about a traumatic incident can help prevent development of a trauma-related disorder. Displaying emotions following a traumatic incident can help prevent development of a trauma-related disorder.

   (N) *NCLEX® Connection: Psychosocial Integrity, Crisis Intervention*

2. **A, C, D. CORRECT:** Manifestations of PTSD include the inability to concentrate on or complete tasks, having recurring nightmares or flashbacks, feeling guilty, and having a negative self-image. A client who has PTSD is reluctant to talk about the traumatic event that triggered the disorder and has an increased startle reflex and hypervigilance.

   (N) *NCLEX® Connection: Psychosocial Integrity, Mental Health Concepts*

3. **D. CORRECT:** The client who has ASD often expresses dissociative manifestations regarding the event, which includes a sense of unreality. The client who has ASD tends to be unable to remember details about the incident and can block the entire incident from memory. The client who has ASD reacts to what is happening with negative emotions (anger, guilt, depression, and anxiety). Elation is an emotion that can occur in clients who have mania. Manifestations of ASD occur immediately to a few days following the event.

   (N) *NCLEX® Connection: Psychosocial Integrity, Mental Health Concepts*

4. **D. CORRECT:** Stating that one's surroundings are far away or unreal in some way is an example of derealization. Feeling that one's body is floating above the ground is an example of depersonalization, in which the person seems to observe their own body from a distance. Having the idea of being targeted in order to be killed and robbed is an example of a paranoid delusion. Being unable to recall any events from the past 2 weeks is an example of amnesia.

   (N) *NCLEX® Connection: Psychosocial Integrity, Mental Health Concepts*

5. **D. CORRECT:** Grounding techniques (stomping the feet, clapping the hands, or touching physical objects) are useful for clients who have a dissociative disorder and are experiencing manifestations of derealization. The client who has dissociative identity disorder displays multiple personalities, while the client who has dissociative fugue has amnesia regarding their identity and past. Avoid flooding the client with information about past events, which can increase the client's level of anxiety. Encourage the client to make decisions regarding routine daily activities in order to promote improved self-esteem and decrease the client's feelings of powerlessness.

   (N) *NCLEX® Connection: Psychosocial Integrity, Mental Health Concepts*

6. **A, C, D. CORRECT:** Concurrent administration of a low-dose of buspirone is an effective measure to manage the adverse effect of paroxetine. Using a mouth guard during sleep can decrease the risk for oral damage resulting from bruxism. Changing to a different class of antianxiety medication that does not have the adverse effect of bruxism is an effective measure. Other SSRIs will also have bruxism as an adverse effect; therefore, this is not an effective measure. Increasing the dose of paroxetine can cause the adverse effect of bruxism to worsen; therefore, this is not an effective measure.

   (N) *NCLEX® Connection: Pharmacological Therapies, Expected Actions/Outcomes*

Active Learning Scenario

A nurse is caring for a client who has post traumatic stress disorder (PTSD) following several months in a military combat situation. Use the Active Learning Template: System Disorder to complete this item.

ALTERATIONS IN HEALTH (DIAGNOSIS): Differentiate PTSD from acute stress disorder (ASD).

EXPECTED FINDINGS: List three subjective and three objective manifestations of PTSD.

NURSING CARE: List three nursing actions for a client who has PTSD.

THERAPEUTIC PROCEDURES: Describe two therapeutic techniques used to treat a client who has PTSD.

Active Learning Scenario Key

Using the ATI Active Learning Template: System Disorder

ALTERATIONS IN HEALTH (DIAGNOSIS)
- Both disorders follow a traumatic incident or multiple experiences that the client perceives as traumatic.
- ASD manifestations occur soon after the incident but subside within 1 month of the trauma.
- PTSD findings can be delayed for weeks or months after the trauma has subsided and continue for months or years, often causing severe social and occupational implications.

EXPECTED FINDINGS
- Subjective manifestations: Client describes dreams and/or flashbacks of the traumatic event; client reports having insomnia; client verbalizes guilt and self-blame.
- Objective manifestations: Hyperactive startle reflexes; manifestations of anxiety (tachycardia, hyperventilation); inability to focus in order to complete a simple task

NURSING CARE
- Monitor for suicidal ideation, and take precautions if it occurs.
- Provide a safe, routine environment for the client.
- Reinforce teaching strategies to decrease anxiety (breathing techniques or music therapy).
- Encourage the client to share feelings.
- Use therapeutic communication techniques to assist a client who has cognitive distortions.

THERAPEUTIC PROCEDURES: Therapeutic techniques for a client who has PTSD include eye movement desensitization and reprocessing (EMDR), group and family therapy, and cognitive behavioral therapy.

(N) *NCLEX® Connection: Psychosocial Integrity, Coping Mechanisms*

M◇ *Online Video: Understanding Major Depression*

UNIT 3   PSYCHOBIOLOGIC DISORDERS

CHAPTER 13 *Depressive Disorders*

Depression is a mood (affective) disorder that is a widespread issue, ranking high among causes of disability.

A client who has depression has a potential risk for suicide, especially if they have a family or personal history of suicide attempts, comorbid anxiety disorder or panic attacks, comorbid substance use disorder or psychosis, poor self-esteem, a lack of social support, or a chronic medical condition.

COMMON COMORBIDITIES

Anxiety disorders: These disorders are comorbid in approximately 70% of clients who have a depressive disorder. This combination makes a client's prognosis poorer, with a higher risk for suicide and disability.

Psychotic disorders (schizophrenia)

Substance use disorders: Clients often use substances in an attempt to relieve manifestations of depression or self-treat mental health disorders.

Eating disorders

Personality disorders

DEPRESSIVE DISORDERS RECOGNIZED BY THE DSM-5-TR

Major depressive disorder (MDD): A single episode or recurrent episodes of unipolar depression (not associated with mood swings from major depression to mania) resulting in a significant change in a client's normal functioning (social, occupational, self-care), accompanied by at least five of the following specific clinical findings, which must occur almost every day for a minimum of 2 weeks and last most of the day
- Depressed mood
- Difficulty sleeping or excessive sleeping
- Indecisiveness
- Decreased ability to concentrate
- Suicidal ideation
- Increase or decrease in motor activity
- Inability to feel pleasure
- Increase or decrease in weight of more than 5% of total body weight over 1 month

A bereavement exclusion was previously used when a client experienced clinical findings of depression within the first 2 months after a significant loss. Now, however, a client can be diagnosed with depression during this time so that needed treatment will not be delayed.

- MDD can be further diagnosed in the DSM-5 with a more specific classification (specifier), including the following.
  - **Psychotic features:** The presence of auditory hallucinations (such as voices telling the client they are sinful) or the presence of delusions (such as the client thinking that they have a fatal disease)
  - **Postpartum onset:** A depressive episode that begins within 4 weeks of childbirth (known as postpartum depression) and can include delusions, which can put the newborn infant at high risk of being harmed by the mother

Seasonal affective disorder (SAD): A form of depression that occurs seasonally, usually during the winter, when there is less daylight. Light therapy is the first-line treatment for SAD.

Persistent depressive disorder (previously known as dysrhythmic disorder): A milder form of depression that usually has an early onset (in childhood or adolescence) and lasts at least 2 years for adults (1 year for children). Persistent depressive disorder contains at least three clinical findings of depression and can, later in life, become major depressive disorder.

Premenstrual dysphoric disorder (PMDD): A depressive disorder associated with the luteal phase of the menstrual cycle. The prevalence of premenstrual dysphoric disorder is 2% to 6% of menstruating clients and causes problems that can be severe enough to interfere with the ability of a client to work or interact with others. Emotional manifestations can include mood swings, irritability, depression, anxiety, feeling of being overwhelmed, and difficulty concentrating. Physical manifestations can include lack of energy, overeating, hyper- or insomnia, breast tenderness, aching, bloating, and weight gain. Treatment includes exercise, diet, and relaxation therapy.

Substance-induced depressive disorder: Clinical findings of depression that are associated with the use of, or withdrawal from, drugs and alcohol

CLIENT CARE

Care of a client who has MDD will mirror the phase of the disease that the client is experiencing. Qᴘᴄᴄ

Acute phase
- Treatment is generally 6 to 12 weeks in duration.
- Potential need for hospitalization
- Reduction of depressive manifestations is the goal of treatment.
- Monitor suicide risk, and implement safety precautions or one-to-one observation as needed.

Continuation phase
- Treatment is generally 4 to 9 months in duration.
- Relapse prevention through education, medication therapy, and psychotherapy is the goal of treatment.

Maintenance phase
- This phase can last for years.
- Prevention of future depressive episodes is the goal of treatment.

DATA COLLECTION

RISK FACTORS

- **Family history and a previous personal history of depression** are the most significant risk factors.
- Depressive disorders are twice as common in **females** than in males.
- Depression is very common among **clients over age 65**, but the disorder is more difficult to recognize in the older adult client and can go untreated. It is important to differentiate between early dementia and depression. Some clinical findings of depression that can look like dementia are memory loss, confusion, and behavioral problems (social isolation or agitation). Clients can seek health care for somatic problems that are manifestations of untreated depression. ⓖ
- **Neurotransmitter deficiencies** (a serotonin deficiency [affects mood, sexual behavior, sleep cycles, hunger, and pain perception] or a norepinephrine deficiency [affects attention and behavior]) can be risk factors for depression. Imbalances of the neurotransmitters norepinephrine, dopamine, acetylcholine, GABA, and possibly glutamate can play a role in the occurrence of depression.

OTHER RISK FACTORS
- Stressful life events
- Presence of a medical illness
- Postpartum period
- Comorbid anxiety or personality disorder
- Comorbid substance use disorder
- Trauma occurring early in life

> Depressive disorders occur throughout all groups of people.
>
> Depression can be the primary disorder or a response to another physical or mental health disorder.

EXPECTED FINDINGS

- Anergia (lack of energy)
- Anhedonia (lack of pleasure in normal activities)
- Anxiety
- Reports of sluggishness (most common) or feeling unable to relax and sit still
- Vegetative findings, which include a change in eating patterns (usually anorexia in MDD; increased intake in persistent depressive disorder and PMDD), change in bowel habits (usually constipation), sleep disturbances, and decreased interest in sexual activity
- Somatic reports (fatigue, gastrointestinal changes, pain)

PHYSICAL ASSESSMENT FINDINGS
- The client most often looks sad with blunted affect.
- The client exhibits poor grooming and lack of hygiene.
- Psychomotor retardation (slowed physical movement, slumped posture) is more common, but psychomotor agitation (restlessness, pacing, finger tapping) can also occur.
- The client becomes socially isolated, showing little or no effort to interact.
- Slowed speech, decreased verbalization, delayed response: The client might seem too tired to speak and can sigh often.

STANDARDIZED SCREENING TOOLS

- Hamilton Depression Scale
- Beck Depression Inventory
- Geriatric Depression Scale (short form) ⓖ
- Zung Self-Rating Depression Scale
- Patient Health Questionnaire-9 (PHQ-9)

PATIENT-CENTERED CARE

NURSING CARE

Milieu therapy

Suicide risk: Determine the client's risk for suicide, and implement appropriate safety precautions.

Self-care: Monitor the client's ability to perform activities of daily living, and encourage independence as much as possible.

Communication: Relate therapeutically to the client who is unable or unwilling to communicate.
- Make time to be with the client, even if they do not speak.
- Make observations rather than asking direct questions, which can cause anxiety in the client. For example, the nurse might say, "I noticed that you attended the unit group meeting today," rather than asking, "Did you enjoy the group meeting?" Give directions in simple, concrete sentences because a client who has depression can have difficulty focusing on and comprehending long sentences. Ⓠ EBP
- Give the client sufficient time to respond when holding a conversation due to a possible delayed response time.

Maintenance of a safe environment

Counseling: This can include individual counseling to assist with the following.
- Problem-solving
- Increasing coping abilities
- Changing negative thinking to positive
- Increasing self-esteem
- Assertiveness training
- Using available community resources

PSYCHOPHARMACOLOGICAL THERAPIES

MEDICATIONS

REINFORCEMENT OF CLIENT TEACHING FOR ALL ANTIDEPRESSANTS
- Do not discontinue medication suddenly. Ⓠs
- Therapeutic effects are not immediate, and it can take several weeks or more to reach full therapeutic benefits.
- Avoid hazardous activities (driving or operating heavy equipment/machinery) due to the potential adverse effect of sedation.
- Notify the provider of any thoughts of suicide.
- Avoid alcohol while taking an antidepressant.

Tricyclic antidepressants

Amitriptyline

CLIENT EDUCATION
- Change positions slowly to minimize dizziness from orthostatic hypotension.
- To minimize anticholinergic effects, chew sugarless gum, eat foods high in fiber, and increase fluid intake to 2 to 3 L/day from food and beverage sources.

Monoamine oxidase inhibitors

Phenelzine

CLIENT EDUCATION
- Due to the risk for hypertensive crisis, avoid foods with tyramine (ripe avocados or figs, fermented or smoked meats, liver, dried or cured fish, most cheeses, some beer and wine, and protein dietary supplements).
- Due to the risk of medication interactions, avoid all medications, including over-the-counter, without first discussing them with the provider.

Atypical antidepressants

Bupropion

CLIENT EDUCATION
- Observe for headache, dry mouth, GI distress, constipation, increased heart rate, nausea, restlessness, or insomnia, and notify the provider if they become intolerable.
- Monitor food intake and weight due to appetite suppression.
- Avoid administering if at risk for seizures.

Selective serotonin reuptake inhibitors

SELECTIVE SEROTONIN REUPTAKE INHIBITORS (SSRIS)

Leading treatment for depression

SELECT PROTOTYPE MEDICATION: Paroxetine

OTHER MEDICATIONS
- Citalopram
- Fluoxetine
- Sertraline

CLIENT EDUCATION

- Adverse effects can include nausea, headache, and central nervous system stimulation (agitation, insomnia, anxiety).
- Be aware that sexual dysfunction can occur, and notify provider if effects are intolerable.
- Observe for manifestations of serotonin syndrome. If any occur, withhold the medication and notify the provider.
- Avoid the concurrent use of St. John's wort, which can increase the risk of serotonin syndrome.
- Follow a healthy diet and exercise regimen because weight gain can occur with long-term use.

PURPOSE

EXPECTED PHARMACOLOGICAL ACTION

- SSRIs selectively inhibit serotonin reuptake, allowing more serotonin to stay at the junction of the neurons.
- SSRIs do not block uptake of dopamine or norepinephrine.
- Paroxetine causes CNS stimulation, which can cause insomnia.
- As SSRIs have a long effective half-life, up to 4 weeks are necessary to produce therapeutic medication levels.

THERAPEUTIC USES Q EBP

SSRI antidepressants are the first-line treatment for panic disorders and trauma- and stressor-related disorders.

Paroxetine
- Generalized anxiety disorder (GAD)
- Panic disorder: decreases both the frequency and intensity of panic attacks, and also prevents anticipatory anxiety about attacks
- Obsessive-compulsive disorder (OCD): reduces manifestations by increasing serotonin
- Social anxiety disorder
- Posttraumatic stress disorder (PTSD)
- Depressive disorders
- Adjustment disorders
- Associated manifestations of dissociative disorders

Sertraline is indicated for panic disorder, OCD, social anxiety disorder, and PTSD.

Citalopram is indicated for panic disorder, OCD, GAD, PTSD, and social anxiety disorder.

Escitalopram is indicated for GAD, OCD, panic disorder, PTSD, and social anxiety disorder.

Fluoxetine is used for panic disorder, social anxiety disorder, OCD, and PTSD.

Fluvoxamine is used for OCD, GAD, social anxiety disorder, and PTSD.

COMPLICATIONS

Early adverse effects

First few days/weeks: nausea, diaphoresis, tremor, fatigue, drowsiness

CLIENT EDUCATION
- Report adverse effects to the provider.
- Take the medication as prescribed.
- These effects should soon subside.
- Avoid driving if these effects occur.

Later adverse effects

After 5 to 6 weeks of therapy: sexual dysfunction (impotence, delayed or absent orgasm, delayed or absent ejaculation, decreased sexual interest), weight gain, headache

CLIENT EDUCATION: Report problems with sexual function (managed with dose reduction, medication holiday, changing medications).

Weight changes

Occurrence of weight loss early in therapy that can be followed by weight gain with long-term treatment

NURSING ACTIONS: Monitor the client's weight.

CLIENT EDUCATION: Follow a well-balanced diet and exercise regularly.

Gastrointestinal bleeding

NURSING ACTIONS: Use cautiously in clients who have a history of gastrointestinal bleed, and ulcers and those taking other medications that affect blood coagulation.

CLIENT EDUCATION: Report indications of bleeding (dark stools, emesis that has the appearance of coffee grounds).

Hyponatremia

More likely in older adult clients taking diuretics Ⓖ

NURSING ACTIONS: Obtain baseline blood sodium, and monitor level periodically throughout treatment.

Serotonin syndrome

Can begin 2 to 72 hr after starting treatment and can be lethal

MANIFESTATIONS
- Confusion, agitation, poor concentration, hostility
- Disorientation, hallucinations, delirium
- Seizures leading to status epilepticus
- Tachycardia leading to cardiovascular shock
- Labile blood pressure
- Diaphoresis
- Fever leading to hyperpyrexia
- Incoordination, hyperreflexia
- Nausea, vomiting, diarrhea, abdominal pain
- Coma leading to apnea (and death in severe cases)

CLIENT EDUCATION: Observe for manifestations. If any occur, withhold the medication and notify the provider.

Bruxism

Grinding and clenching of teeth, usually during sleep

NURSING ACTIONS
Report bruxism to the provider, who may:
- Switch the client to another class of medication
- Treat bruxism with low-dose buspirone

CLIENT EDUCATION: Use a mouth guard during sleep.

Withdrawal syndrome

Nausea, sensory disturbances, anxiety, tremor, malaise, unease

CLIENT EDUCATION
- After a long period of use, taper the medication slowly according to a prescribed tapered dosing schedule to avoid withdrawal effects.
- Avoid abrupt discontinuation of the medication.

CONTRAINDICATIONS/PRECAUTIONS Ⓠs

- Paroxetine is a teratogenic medication. Other SSRIs pose less risk during pregnancy.
- SSRIs are contraindicated in clients taking MAOIs or TCAs.
- Clients should avoid alcohol while taking SSRIs.
- Use cautiously in clients who have liver and renal dysfunction, seizure disorders, or a history of gastrointestinal bleeding.
- Use SSRIs cautiously in clients who have bipolar disorder, due to the risk for mania. Ⓠs

INTERACTIONS

Concurrent use of TCAs, MAOIs, or St. John's wort can cause serotonin syndrome.
NURSING ACTIONS
- Discontinue MAOIs 14 days prior to starting an SSRI.
- Fluoxetine (SSRI) should be discontinued 5 weeks before starting an MAOI.
- Advise the client against concurrent use of TCAs or St. John's wort with SSRIs.

Concurrent use with warfarin can displace warfarin from bound protein and result in increased warfarin levels.
NURSING ACTIONS
- Monitor prothrombin time (PT) and INR levels.
- Monitor for indications of bleeding and the need for dosage adjustment.

Concurrent use with TCAs and lithium can result in increased levels of these medications.
CLIENT EDUCATION: Avoid concurrent use.

Concurrent use with NSAIDs and anticoagulants can further suppress platelet aggregation, thereby increasing the risk of bleeding.
CLIENT EDUCATION: Monitor for indications of bleeding (bruising, hematuria) and notify the provider if they occur.

NURSING ADMINISTRATION

CLIENT EDUCATION
- SSRIs may be taken with food. Sleep disturbances are minimized by taking the medication in the morning. ⓆEBP
- Take the medication on a daily basis to establish therapeutic plasma levels.
- It can take up to 4 weeks to achieve therapeutic effects.

Serotonin norepinephrine reuptake inhibitors

SELECT PROTOTYPE MEDICATION: Venlafaxine

OTHER MEDICATIONS: Duloxetine

NURSING ACTIONS
- Adverse effects include nausea, insomnia, weight gain, diaphoresis, and sexual dysfunction.
- Caution in administering to clients who have a history of hypertension

PURPOSE

EXPECTED PHARMACOLOGICAL ACTION: Inhibit the uptake of serotonin and norepinephrine; minimal inhibition of dopamine

THERAPEUTIC USES: Used for major depression, panic disorders, and generalized anxiety disorder

COMPLICATIONS

Headache, nausea, agitation, anxiety, dry mouth, and sleep disturbances

NURSING ACTIONS: Report adverse effects to the provider.

Hyponatremia, especially in older adult clients taking diuretics

NURSING ACTIONS: Obtain baseline blood sodium, and monitor level periodically throughout treatment.

Anorexia resulting in weight loss

NURSING ACTIONS: Monitor the client's weight. Q PCC

CLIENT EDUCATION: Follow a well-balanced diet and exercise regularly.

Hypertension

NURSING ACTIONS: Monitor for increases in blood pressure.

Sexual dysfunction

NURSING ACTIONS: Report problems with sexual function (managed with dose reduction, medication holiday, changing medications).

CONTRAINDICATIONS/PRECAUTIONS

- SNRIs are teratogenic.
- SNRIs are contraindicated in clients taking MAOIs.
- Duloxetine should not be used in clients who have hepatic disease or in those who consume large amounts of alcohol.

CLIENT EDUCATION
- Avoid abrupt cessation of the medication.
- Avoid alcohol while taking SNRIs.

13.1 Case study

Scenario introduction

Maria: "I am concerned about my friend Cary, who seems severely depressed. That is why I brought them to the clinic today. Maybe you can give them some medicine to help?"

Nurse Juan: "Thank you for helping Cary come to the clinic. The provider will assess them soon."

Scene 1

Nurse Juan: "Tell me about the symptoms you have been having, Cary."

Cary: "I have no energy, no interest in doing anything, and extreme fatigue, and I cry a lot. (The client has a flat affect, makes no eye contact, has slowed speech, and has poor hygiene.)"

Scene 2

Nurse Juan: "Based on the Hamilton Depression Scale score of 23, you are experiencing moderate depression. How long have you had these feelings?"

Cary: "I have been like this for about 3 months now. I'm just depressed. I lost my job, and my best friend died two months ago. I don't know what else to do. I don't want to be a burden to anyone."

Scenario conclusion

The nurse and provider review the assessment findings together and develop a plan of care for the client.

Case study exercises

1. The nurse is discussing manifestations of depressive disorder with the client. Which of the following statements should the nurse make?
   A. "You mentioned that you feel depressed. Tell me about what those feelings are like for you."
   B. "Have you tried to get another job?"
   C. "Did you go to your friend's service after they died?"
   D. "Do you feel like talking about being depressed?"

2. The nurse should instruct the client to avoid food containing tyramine because the provider has prescribed phenelzine. Which of these foods contain tyramine? (Select all that apply.)
   A. Ripe avocados
   B. Liver
   C. Bread
   D. Smoked meats
   E. Bananas

INTERACTIONS

Concurrent use of MAOIs and St. John's wort can cause serotonin syndrome.
- NURSING ACTIONS: Discontinue MAOIs 14 days prior to starting an SNRI.
- CLIENT EDUCATION: Avoid concurrent use of St. John's wort along with SNRIs.

CNS depression with alcohol, opioids, antihistamines, sedative/hypnotics
NURSING ACTIONS: Avoid concurrent use.

Concurrent use with NSAIDs and anticoagulants can further suppress platelet aggregation, thereby increasing the risk of bleeding.
CLIENT EDUCATION: Monitor for indications of bleeding (bruising, hematuria) and notify the provider if they occur.

NURSING ADMINISTRATION

Duloxetine should not be used in clients who have hepatic disease or in those who consume large amounts of alcohol.

CLIENT EDUCATION
- Avoid abrupt cessation of the medication. ○EBP
- SNRIs may be taken with food.
- Take the medication on a daily basis to establish therapeutic plasma levels.
- Medication can take up to 4 weeks to achieve therapeutic effects.

ALTERNATIVE OR COMPLEMENTARY THERAPIES

St. John's wort

A plant product (*Hypericum perforatum*), not regulated by the U.S. Food and Drug Administration, is taken by some individuals to relieve manifestations of mild depression.

NURSING ACTIONS
- Adverse effects include photosensitivity, skin rash, rapid heart rate, gastrointestinal distress, and abdominal pain.
- St. John's wort can increase or reduce levels of some medications if taken concurrently. The client should inform the provider if taking St. John's wort.

> ! Medication interactions: Potentially fatal serotonin syndrome can result if St. John's wort is taken with SSRIs or other types of antidepressants. Foods containing tyramine should be avoided.

Light therapy

- First-line treatment for SAD, light therapy inhibits nocturnal secretion of melatonin.
- Exposure of the face to 10,000-lux light box 30 min/day, once or in two divided doses

THERAPEUTIC PROCEDURES

Electroconvulsive therapy

Can be useful for some clients who have a depressive disorder and are unresponsive to other treatments

NURSING ACTIONS: A specially trained nurse is responsible for monitoring the client before and after this therapy.

Transcranial magnetic stimulation

Uses electromagnetic stimulation (MRI strength magnetic pulsation) to stimulate focal areas of cerebral cortex. It is indicated for depressive disorders that are resistant to other forms of treatment.

Vagus nerve stimulation

Uses an implanted device that stimulates the vagus nerve. It can be used for clients who have depression that is resistant to antidepressant medications.

Deep brain stimulation

A treatment that surgically implants electrodes into the brain to stimulate underactive regions. It is reserved for clients who have tried many other treatments that have failed. The nurse should use standard postoperative care for these clients.

INTERPROFESSIONAL CARE

Psychotherapy by a trained therapist can include individual cognitive-behavioral therapy (CBT), interpersonal therapy (IPT), group therapy, and family therapy.
- CBT assists the client to identify and change negative behavior and thought patterns.
- IPT encourages the client to focus on personal relationships that contribute to the depressive disorder.

CLIENT EDUCATION

Continuation phase followed by maintenance phase
- Review manifestations of depression with the client and family members in order to identify relapse.
- Reinforce intended effects and potential adverse effects of medication.
- Explain the benefits of adherence to therapy.
- Thirty minutes of exercise daily for 3 to 5 days each week improves clinical findings of depression and can help to prevent relapse. Even shorter intervals of exercise are helpful. Exercise should be regarded as an adjunct to other therapies for the client who has major depressive disorder. ○EBP

NURSING EVALUATION OF MEDICATION EFFECTIVENESS

Depending on therapeutic intent, effectiveness is evidenced by the following.
- Verbalized feeling of less anxiety
- Description of improved mood
- Improved memory retrieval
- Maintenance of a normal sleep pattern
- Greater ability to participate in social and occupational interactions
- Improved ability to cope with manifestations and identified stressors
- Ability to perform activities of daily living
- Report of increased well-being

Active Learning Scenario

A nurse working in an acute mental health facility is collecting data collection from a client who has major depressive disorder (MDD). Use the *ATI Active Learning Template: System Disorder* to complete this item.

ALTERATIONS IN HEALTH (DIAGNOSIS)

EXPECTED FINDINGS: Identify at least four expected findings.

NURSING CARE: Describe an appropriate communication technique to relate therapeutically with this client.

Application Exercises

1. A charge nurse is discussing the care of a client who has major depressive disorder (MDD) with a newly licensed nurse. Which of the following statements by the newly licensed nurse indicates an understanding of the teaching?
   A. "Care during the continuation phase focuses on treating continued manifestations of MDD."
   B. "The treatment of MDD during the maintenance phase lasts for 6 to 12 weeks."
   C. "The client is at greatest risk for suicide during the first weeks of an MDD episode."
   D. "Medication and psychotherapy are most effective during the acute phase of MDD."

2. A nurse is caring for a client who has major depressive disorder. Which of the following should the nurse identify as a risk factor for depression? (Select all that apply.)
   A. Male sex
   B. History of chronic bronchitis
   C. Recent death in client's family
   D. Family history of depression
   E. Personal history of panic disorder

3. A nurse is interviewing a client who has a new diagnosis of persistent depressive disorder. Which of the following findings should the nurse expect?
   A. Wide fluctuations in mood
   B. Report of a minimum of five clinical findings of depression
   C. Presence of manifestations for at least 2 years
   D. Inflated sense of self-esteem

4. A nurse working on an acute mental health unit is admitting a client who has major depressive disorder and comorbid anxiety disorder. Which of the following actions is the nurse's priority?
   A. Place the client on one-to-one observation.
   B. Assist the client to perform ADLs.
   C. Encourage the client to participate in counseling.
   D. Reinforce education about medication adverse effects.

5. A nurse is monitoring a client 4 hr after the client has received an initial dose of fluoxetine. Which of the following findings should the nurse report to the provider as indications of serotonin syndrome? (Select all that apply.)
   A. Hypothermia
   B. Hallucinations
   C. Muscular flaccidity
   D. Diaphoresis
   E. Agitation

Active Learning Scenario Key

Using the ATI Active Learning Template: System Disorder

ALTERATIONS IN HEALTH (DIAGNOSIS): MDD is a single episode or recurrent episodes of unipolar depression resulting in a significant change in a client's normal functioning (social, occupational, self-care), accompanied by at least five clinical findings of MDD, which must occur almost every day for a minimum of 2 weeks and last most of the day.

EXPECTED FINDINGS
- Depressed mood
- Difficulty sleeping or excessive sleeping
- Indecisiveness
- Decreased ability to concentrate
- Suicidal ideation
- Increase or decrease in motor activity
- Inability to feel pleasure (anhedonia)
- Increase or decrease in weight of more than 5% of total body weight over 1 month

NURSING CARE
- Make time to be with the client even if they don't speak.
- Communicate with observations rather than asking direct questions.
- Give directions in simple, concrete sentences.
- Allow the client sufficient time to verbally respond.

Ⓝ *NCLEX® Connection: Psychosocial Integrity, Mental Health Concepts*

Case Study Exercises Key

1. A. **CORRECT:** The nurse should use open communication techniques to encourage the client to express openly how they are feeling. The other statements are closed-ended and impede further communication.

   Ⓝ *NCLEX® Connection: Pharmacological Therapies, Adverse Effects/Contraindications/Side Effects/Interactions*

2. A, B, D. **CORRECT:** Ripe avocados, liver, and smoked meats contain tyramine. The nurse should instruct the client to avoid foods containing tyramine.

   Ⓝ *NCLEX® Connection: Pharmacological Therapies, Adverse Effects/Contraindications/Side Effects/Interactions*

Application Exercises Key

1. C. **CORRECT:** The client is at greatest risk for suicide during the acute phase of MDD. The focus of the continuation phase is relapse prevention. Treatment of manifestations occurs during the acute phase of MDD. The maintenance phase of treatment for MDD can last for 1 year or more. Medication therapy and psychotherapy are used during the continuation phase to prevent relapse of MDD.

   Ⓝ *NCLEX® Connection: Psychosocial Integrity, Mental Health Concepts*

2. B, C, D, E. **CORRECT:** Females are twice as likely as males to experience a depressive disorder. Depressive disorders are more common in a client who has a chronic medical condition. Depressive disorders are more likely to occur in a client who is experiencing a high amount of stress (when grieving the death of a family member). Depressive disorders are more likely to occur in a client who has a family history of depression. A history of an anxiety or personality disorder increases a client's risk for depressive disorder.

   Ⓝ *NCLEX® Connection: Health Promotion and Maintenance, Health Promotion/Disease Prevention*

3. C. **CORRECT:** Manifestations of persistent depressive disorder last for at least 2 years in adults. Wide fluctuations in mood are associated with bipolar disorder. MDD contains a minimum of three clinical findings of depression. A decreased, rather than inflated, sense of self-esteem is associated with persistent depressive disorder.

   Ⓝ *NCLEX® Connection: Psychosocial Integrity, Mental Health Concepts*

4. A. **CORRECT:** The greatest risk for a client who has MDD and comorbid anxiety is injury due to self-harm. The highest priority intervention is placing the client on one-to-one observation. The client who has MDD can require assistance with ADLs. However, this does not address the greatest risk to the client and is therefore not the priority intervention. Encourage the client who has MDD to participate in counseling. However, this does not address the greatest risk to the client and is therefore not the priority intervention. Teaching the client who has MDD about medication adverse effects does not address the greatest risk to the client and is therefore not the priority intervention.

   Ⓝ *NCLEX® Connection: Psychosocial Integrity, Crisis Intervention*

5. B, D, E. **CORRECT:** Hallucinations are an indication of serotonin syndrome. Diaphoresis is an indication of serotonin syndrome. Agitation is an indication of serotonin syndrome. Fever, rather than hypothermia, is an indication of serotonin syndrome. Muscle tremors, rather than flaccidity, are an indication of serotonin syndrome.

   Ⓝ *NCLEX® Connection: Pharmacological Therapies, Adverse Effects/Contraindications/Adverse Effects/Interactions*

UNIT 3   PSYCHOBIOLOGIC DISORDERS

CHAPTER 14 *Bipolar Disorders*

Bipolar disorders are mood disorders with recurrent episodes of depression and mania.

Bipolar disorders usually emerge in early adulthood, but early-onset bipolar disorder can be diagnosed in pediatric clients. Because manifestations can mimic expected findings of attention deficit hyperactivity disorder (ADHD), it is more difficult to monitor and diagnose bipolar disorders in children than in other client age groups.

Periods of normal functioning alternate with periods of illness, though some clients are not able to maintain full occupational and social functioning. Clients can exhibit psychotic, paranoid, and/or bizarre behavior during periods of mania.

CLIENT CARE

Care of a client who has bipolar disorder will mirror the behaviors of the disease that the client is manifesting.

Acute phase
- Hospitalization can be required.
- Reduction of mania and client safety are the goals of treatment.
- Risk of harm to self or others is determined.
- One-to-one supervision can be indicated for client safety. Qs

Continuation phase
- Treatment is generally 4 to 9 months in duration.
- Relapse prevention through education, medication adherence, and psychotherapy is the goal of treatment.

Maintenance phase
- Treatment generally continues throughout the client's lifetime.
- Prevention of future manic episodes is the goal of treatment.

BEHAVIORS SHOWN WITH BIPOLAR DISORDERS

Mania: An abnormally elevated mood, which can also be described as expansive or irritable; usually requires hospitalization. Manic episodes last at least 1 week. (See the **DATA COLLECTION** section in this chapter for specific findings.)

Hypomania: A less severe episode of mania that lasts at least 4 days, accompanied by three or more manifestations of mania. Hospitalization is not required, and the client who has hypomania is less impaired. Hypomania can progress to mania.

Rapid cycling: Four or more episodes of hypomania or acute mania within 1 year and associated with increased recurrence rate and resistance to treatment

TYPES OF BIPOLAR DISORDERS

Bipolar I disorder: The client has at least one episode of mania alternating with major depression.

Bipolar II disorder: The client has one or more hypomanic episodes alternating with major depressive episodes.

Cyclothymic disorder: The client has at least 2 years of repeated hypomanic manifestations that do not meet the criteria for hypomanic episodes alternating with minor depressive episodes.

COMORBIDITIES

- Substance use disorder
- Anxiety disorders
- Borderline personality disorder
- Oppositional defiant disorder
- Social phobia and specific phobias
- Seasonal affective disorder
- Attention deficit hyperactivity disorder
- Migraines
- Metabolic syndrome

DATA COLLECTION

RISK FACTORS

Genetics: Having an immediate family member who has a bipolar disorder

Physiological: Neurobiologic and neuroendocrine disorders

Environmental: Increased stress in the environment can trigger mania and depression and increase risk for severe manifestations in genetically-susceptible children.

RELAPSE

- Use of substances (alcohol, cocaine, caffeine) can lead to an episode of mania.
- Sleep disturbances can come before, be associated with, or be brought on by an episode of mania.
- Psychological stressors can trigger an episode of mania.

EXPECTED FINDINGS

MANIC CHARACTERISTICS

- Labile mood with euphoria
- Agitation and irritability
- Restlessness
- Dislike of interference and intolerance of criticism
- Increase in talking and activity
- Flight of ideas: rapid, continuous speech with sudden and frequent topic change
- Grandiose view of self and abilities (grandiosity)
- Impulsivity: spending money, giving away money or possessions
- Demanding and manipulative behavior
- Distractibility and decreased attention span
- Poor judgment
- Attention-seeking behavior: flashy dress and makeup, inappropriate behavior
- Impairment in social and occupational functioning
- Decreased sleep
- Neglect of ADLs, including nutrition and hydration
- Possible presence of delusions and hallucinations
- Denial of illness

DEPRESSIVE CHARACTERISTICS

- Flat, blunted, labile affect
- Tearfulness, crying
- Lack of energy
- Anhedonia: loss of pleasure and lack of interest in activities, hobbies, sexual activity
- Physical reports of discomfort/pain
- Difficulty concentrating, focusing, problem-solving
- Self-destructive behavior, including suicidal ideation
- Decrease in personal hygiene
- Loss or increase in appetite and/or sleep, disturbed sleep
- Psychomotor retardation or agitation

STANDARDIZED SCREENING TOOL

Altman Self Rating Mania Scale (ASRM): A standardized tool that assesses the client's placement on the continuum from depression to mania and is useful for the management and treatment of the client.

PATIENT-CENTERED CARE

NURSING CARE

The care of the client is based on the behaviors of bipolar disorder that the client is manifesting. Nursing care is provided throughout this process.

Acute manic episode

Focus is on safety and maintaining physical health. Qs

THERAPEUTIC MILIEU (within acute care mental health facility)

- Provide a safe environment during the acute phase.
- Monitor the client regularly for suicidal thoughts, intentions, and escalating behavior.
- Decrease stimulation without isolating the client if possible. Be aware of noise, music, television, and other clients, all of which can lead to an escalation of the client's behavior. In certain cases, seclusion might be the only way to safely decrease stimulation for the client.
- Follow agency protocols for providing client protection (restraints, seclusion, one-to-one observation) if a threat of self-injury or injury to others exists.
- Implement frequent rest periods.
- Assist with providing outlets for physical activity. Do not involve the client in activities that last a long time or that require a high level of concentration and/or detailed instructions.
- Protect client from poor judgment and impulsive behavior, such as giving money away and sexual indiscretions.
- Remove potentially dangerous items (belts, shoe-strings, perfume/cologne) from client.

MAINTENANCE OF SELF-CARE NEEDS

- Monitoring sleep, fluid intake, and nutrition.
- Providing portable, nutritious food because the client might not be able to sit down to eat.
- Supervising choice of clothes.
- Giving step-by-step reminders for hygiene and dress.

14.1 Case study

Scenario introduction

Spouse Liz and partner Anna present to the mental health facility.

Scene 1

Liz: "My spouse has been spending excessively over the past two months. She is flirting with everyone she sees. One minute, she is singing loudly and the next, screaming and mad. She talks rapidly and nonstop, and she never sits down or sleeps at all. She stopped taking the medication the doctor gave her 3 months ago because she said it slows her down."

Scene 2

Nurse Charlie: "Good morning to you both. How may I help you today?"

Anna: "I am not taking the medicine they had me on because it makes me do everything so slow. Have you ever played cards, done your makeup, swam in the creek, picked flowers, and baked a cake for your birthday?"

Nurse Charlie: "Anna, what medication did the doctor prescribe you?"

Anna: "I need to see the Chief of Staff because the president is on the way to see me. I need the room you have for all your VIP: VERY IMPORTANT PEOPLE! Would you like a signed autographed picture of me? I have a book in the car. I can get Liz to get you it so you'll never forget me."

Scenario conclusion

Nurse Charlie escorts Anna and Liz to a room for the provider to evaluate the client. Anna continues to talk loudly, will not sit down, and is constantly moving around the room and moving things around on the desk.

Case study exercises

1. List the subjective data the client exhibits.

2. List interventions the nurse should take.

COMMUNICATION

- Use a calm, matter-of-fact, specific approach.
- Give concise explanations.
- Provide for consistency with expectations and limit-setting.
- Avoid power struggles, and do not react personally to the client's comments.
- Listen to and act on legitimate client grievances.
- Reinforce nonmanipulative behaviors.
- Use therapeutic communication techniques.

THERAPEUTIC PROCEDURES

Electroconvulsive therapy (ECT): Can be used to moderate extreme manic behavior, especially when pharmacological therapy (lithium) has not worked. Clients who are suicidal or those who have rapid cycling can also benefit from ECT.

COMPLICATIONS

Physical exhaustion and possible death: A client in a true manic state usually will not stop moving, and does not eat, drink, or sleep. This can become a medical emergency. ◯EBP

NURSING ACTIONS

- Prevent client self-harm.
- Decrease client's physical activity.
- Ensure adequate fluid and food intake.
- Promote an adequate amount of sleep each night.
- Assist the client with self-care needs.
- Manage medication appropriately.

CLIENT EDUCATION

- Case management to provide follow-up for the client and the family ◯TC
- Group, family, and individual psychotherapy (cognitive-behavior therapy) to improve problem-solving and interpersonal skills

Health teaching

- The chronicity of the disorder requiring long-term pharmacological and psychological support
- Benefits of psychotherapy and support groups to prevent relapse
- Indications of impending relapse and ways to manage the crisis
- Precipitating factors of relapse (sleep disturbance, use of alcohol or caffeine)
- Importance of maintaining a regular sleep, meal, and activity pattern
- Medication administration and adherence

Mood stabilizers

SELECT PROTOTYPE MEDICATION: Lithium carbonate

PURPOSE

EXPECTED PHARMACOLOGICAL ACTION
- Lithium produces neurochemical changes in the brain, including serotonin receptor blockade.
- There is evidence that lithium decreases neuronal atrophy and/or increases neuronal growth.

THERAPEUTIC USES: Lithium is used in the treatment of bipolar disorders. Lithium controls episodes of acute mania, helps to prevent the return of mania or depression, and decreases the incidence of suicide.

COMPLICATIONS

CLIENT EDUCATION: Some adverse effects resolve within a few weeks of starting the medication. ◯s

Gastrointestinal distress

Nausea, diarrhea, abdominal pain

NURSING ACTIONS
- Advise the client that GI distress is usually transient.
- Administer medication with meals or milk.

Fine hand tremors

Can interfere with purposeful motor skills and can be exacerbated by factors (stress and caffeine)

NURSING ACTIONS
- Administer beta-adrenergic blocking agents (propranolol).
- Adjust dosage to be as low as possible; give in divided doses; or use long-acting formulations.
- Advise the client to report an increase in tremors, which could be a manifestation of lithium toxicity.

Polyuria, mild thirst

NURSING ACTIONS: Use a potassium-sparing diuretic (spironolactone).

CLIENT EDUCATION: Maintain adequate fluid intake by consuming at least 1.5 to 3 L/day fluid from beverages and food sources.

Weight gain

NURSING ACTIONS: Assist the client to follow a healthy diet and regular exercise regimen.

Renal toxicity

NURSING ACTIONS
- Monitor I&O.
- Adjust dosage, and keep dose at the lowest level necessary.
- Assess baseline BUN and creatinine, and monitor kidney function periodically.

Goiter and hypothyroidism

With long-term treatment

NURSING ACTIONS
- Obtain baseline T3, T4, and TSH levels prior to starting treatment, and then annually.
- Administer levothyroxine.

CLIENT EDUCATION: Monitor for indications of hypothyroidism (cold, dry skin; decreased heart rate; weight gain).

Bradydysrhythmias, hypotension, and electrolyte imbalances

CLIENT EDUCATION: Maintain adequate fluid and sodium intake.

Lithium toxicity

Common adverse effects
- LITHIUM LEVEL: Less than 1.5 mEq/L
- MANIFESTATIONS: Diarrhea, nausea, vomiting, thirst, polyuria, muscle weakness, fine hand tremors, slurred speech, lethargy
- NURSING ACTIONS: Instruct the client that manifestations at low levels often improve over time.

Early indications
- LITHIUM LEVEL: 1.5 to 2.0 mEq/L
- MANIFESTATIONS: Mental confusion, sedation, poor coordination, coarse tremors, and ongoing GI distress, including nausea, vomiting, and diarrhea
- NURSING ACTIONS
  - Instruct the client to withhold the medication, and notify the provider.
  - Administer new dosage based on blood lithium and sodium levels.
  - Excretion can need to be promoted.

Advanced indications
- LITHIUM LEVEL: 2.0 to 2.5 mEq/L
- MANIFESTATIONS: Extreme polyuria of dilute urine, tinnitus, giddiness, jerking movements, blurred vision, ataxia, seizures, severe hypotension and stupor leading to coma, and possible death from respiratory complications
- NURSING ACTIONS
  - Administer an emetic to alert clients, or administer gastric lavage.
  - Urea, mannitol, or aminophylline may be prescribed to increase the rate of excretion.

Severe toxicity
- LITHIUM LEVEL: Greater than 2.5 mEq/L
- MANIFESTATIONS: Rapid progression of manifestations leading to coma and death
- Nursing actions: Hemodialysis can be warranted.

CONTRAINDICATIONS/PRECAUTIONS

- Lithium is a Pregnancy Risk Category D medication. It is considered teratogenic, especially during the first trimester of pregnancy.
- Discourage clients from breastfeeding if lithium therapy is necessary.
- Lithium is contraindicated in clients who have severe renal or cardiac disease, hypovolemia, and schizophrenia.
- Use cautiously in older adult clients and clients who have thyroid disease, seizure disorder, or diabetes. Qs

INTERACTIONS

Diuretics

Sodium is excreted with the use of diuretics. With decreased blood sodium, lithium excretion is decreased, which can lead to toxicity.
- NURSING ACTIONS: Monitor for indications of toxicity.
- CLIENT EDUCATION
  - Observe for indications of toxicity and to notify the provider.
  - Maintain a diet adequate in sodium, and drink 1.5 to 3 L/day of water.

NSAIDs

Concurrent use increases renal reabsorption of lithium, leading to toxicity.
- NURSING ACTIONS
  - Avoid use of NSAIDs to prevent toxic accumulation of lithium.
  - Use aspirin as a mild analgesic, as it does not lead to toxicity.

Anticholinergics (antihistamines, tricyclic antidepressants)

Abdominal discomfort can result from anticholinergic-induced urinary retention and polyuria.
CLIENT EDUCATION: Avoid medications that have anticholinergic effects.

NURSING ADMINISTRATION

- Monitor plasma lithium levels while undergoing treatment. At initiation of treatment, monitor levels every 2 to 3 days until stable and then every 1 to 3 months. Closely monitor levels after any dosage change. Lithium blood levels should be obtained in the morning, 10 to 12 hr after last dose.
  - During initial treatment of a manic episode, higher levels can be required (1 to 1.5 mEq/L).
  - Maintenance level range is 0.6 to 1.2 mEq/L.
- Older adult clients are at an increased risk for toxicity and require more frequent monitoring of blood lithium levels. ©
- Care for a client who has advanced or severe lithium toxicity should take place in an acute care setting with supportive measures provided. Hemodialysis can be indicated.

- Advise the client that effects begin within 5 to 7 days.
- Maximum benefits might not be seen for 2 to 3 weeks.
- Advise the client to take lithium as prescribed. This medication must be administered in 2 to 3 doses daily due to a short half-life. Taking lithium with food will help decrease GI distress.
- Encourage the client to adhere to laboratory appointments needed to monitor lithium effectiveness and adverse effects. Emphasize the high risk of toxicity is high due to the narrow therapeutic range. Qs
- Provide nutritional counseling. Stress the importance of adequate fluid and sodium intake.
- Instruct the client to monitor for indications of toxicity and when to contact the provider. The client should withhold the medication and seek medical attention if experiencing diarrhea, vomiting, or excessive sweating.

Mood-stabilizing antiepileptic medications

SELECT PROTOTYPE MEDICATIONS
- Carbamazepine
- Valproate
- Lamotrigine

PURPOSE

EXPECTED PHARMACOLOGICAL ACTION
Antiepileptic medications help treat and manage bipolar disorder through various mechanisms.
- Slowing the entrance of sodium and calcium back into the neuron, thus extending the time it takes for the nerve to return to its active state
- Potentiating the inhibitory effects of gamma butyric acid (GABA)
- Inhibiting glutamic acid (glutamate), which in turn suppresses central nervous system (CNS) excitation QEBP

THERAPEUTIC USES: These medications are used to treat and prevent relapse of manic and depressive episodes. They are particularly useful for clients who have mixed mania and rapid-cycling bipolar disorders.

COMPLICATIONS

CARBAMAZEPINE

Minimal effect on cognitive function

CNS effects

- Nystagmus
- Double vision
- Vertigo
- Staggering gait
- Headache

NURSING ACTIONS
- Administer in low doses initially, and then gradually increase dosage.
- Administer dose at bedtime.

CLIENT EDUCATION: Effects should subside within a few weeks.

Blood dyscrasias

Leukopenia, anemia, thrombocytopenia

NURSING ACTIONS
- Obtain baseline CBC and platelets. Perform ongoing monitoring of these.
- Observe for indications of thrombocytopenia, including bruising and bleeding of gums.
- Monitor for indications of infection (fever or lethargy).

CLIENT EDUCATION: Notify the provider if indications of blood dyscrasias are present.

Teratogenesis

CLIENT EDUCATION: Avoid use in pregnancy.

Hypoosmolarity

Promotes secretion of antidiuretic hormone, which inhibits water excretion by the kidneys, and places the client who has heart failure at risk for fluid overload

NURSING ACTIONS
- Monitor blood sodium.
- Monitor for edema, decrease in urine output, and hypertension.

Skin disorders

Includes dermatitis, rash (Stevens-Johnson syndrome)

NURSING ACTIONS: Treat mild reactions with anti-inflammatory or antihistamine medications.

CLIENT EDUCATION
- Withhold the medication and notify the provider if Stevens-Johnson syndrome occurs.
- Wear sunscreen to reduce chance of skin disorders.

LAMOTRIGINE

Double or blurred vision, dizziness, headache, nausea, vomiting

CLIENT EDUCATION: Avoid performing activities that require concentration or visual acuity. Qs

Serious skin rashes

Includes Stevens-Johnson syndrome

CLIENT EDUCATION: Withhold the medication, and notify the provider if a rash occurs. To minimize risk of serious rash, start with a low dose and slowly increase it.

VALPROATE

GI effects (nausea, vomiting, indigestion)

CLIENT EDUCATION
- These effects are generally self-limiting.
- Take medication with food, or switch to enteric-coated formulations.

Hepatotoxicity

Evidenced by anorexia, nausea, vomiting, fatigue, abdominal pain, jaundice

NURSING ACTIONS
- Assess baseline liver function, and monitor liver function regularly (minimum of every 2 months during the first 6 months of treatment).
- Avoid using in children younger than 2 years old.
- Administer the lowest effective dose.

CLIENT EDUCATION: Observe for indications of hepatotoxicity and notify the provider immediately if they occur.

Pancreatitis

Evidenced by nausea, vomiting, abdominal pain

NURSING ACTIONS
- Monitor amylase levels.
- Discontinue the medication if pancreatitis develops.

CLIENT EDUCATION: Observe for manifestations of pancreatitis and to notify the provider immediately if they occur.

Thrombocytopenia

NURSING ACTIONS: Monitor platelet counts.

CLIENT EDUCATION: Observe for indications (bruising), and notify the provider if these occur.

Teratogenesis

CLIENT EDUCATION
- Avoid use during pregnancy.
- If considering pregnancy, discuss other treatment options with the provider.

Weight gain

CLIENT EDUCATION: Follow a healthy diet and regular exercise regimen.

CONTRAINDICATIONS/PRECAUTIONS

- These medications are Pregnancy Risk Category D medications. They can result in birth defects.
- Carbamazepine is contraindicated in clients who have bone marrow suppression or bleeding disorders.
- Monitor plasma levels of valproate and carbamazepine while undergoing treatment.
  - The therapeutic blood level range for carbamazepine is 4 to 12 mcg/mL.
  - The therapeutic blood level range for valproic acid is 50 to 120 mcg/mL.
- Lamotrigine needs to be slowly titrated to prevent adverse effects.

INTERACTIONS

CARBAMAZEPINE

Oral contraceptives, warfarin: Concurrent use of carbamazepine causes a decrease in the effects of these medications due to stimulation of hepatic and drug-metabolizing enzymes.
- NURSING ACTIONS: Monitor for therapeutic effects of warfarin. Dosage can need to be adjusted.
- CLIENT EDUCATION: Use an alternate form of birth control.

Grapefruit juice inhibits metabolism of carbamazepine, thereby increasing blood levels of the medication.
CLIENT EDUCATION: Avoid intake of grapefruit juice.

Concurrent use of other anticonvulsants decreases the effects of carbamazepine by stimulating metabolism.
NURSING ACTIONS: Monitor carbamazepine levels, and adjust dosages as prescribed.

LAMOTRIGINE

Carbamazepine, phenytoin, phenobarbital: Concurrent use decreases the effect of lamotrigine.
NURSING ACTIONS: Monitor for therapeutic effects, and adjust dosages as prescribed.

Concurrent use of valproate inhibits drug-metabolizing enzymes, thereby increasing the half-life of lamotrigine.
NURSING ACTIONS: Monitor for adverse effects, and adjust dosages as prescribed.

Concurrent use of oral contraceptives decreases the effectiveness of both medications.
CLIENT EDUCATION: Use an alternate form of birth control.

VALPROATE

Concurrent use of other anticonvulsants affects blood levels of valproate.
NURSING ACTIONS: Monitor valproate levels, and adjust dosages as prescribed.

NURSING EVALUATION OF MEDICATION EFFECTIVENESS

Depending on therapeutic intent, effectiveness can be evidenced by the following.

- Relief of acute manic manifestations (flight of ideas, excessive talking, agitation) or depressive manifestations (fatigue, poor appetite, psychomotor retardation)
- Verbalization of improvement in mood
- Ability to perform ADLs
- Improved sleeping and eating habits
- Appropriate interaction with peers

Antipsychotics

- Lurasidone, olanzapine, quetiapine, aripiprazole, risperidone, asenapine, cariprazine, and ziprasidone are useful during acute mania with or without valproate or lithium.
- Ziprasidone, olanzapine, and aripiprazole can be used long-term as prophylaxis against mood episodes.
- Lurasidone is approved for bipolar depression.

Application Exercises

1. A nurse is discussing relapse prevention with a client who has bipolar disorder. Which of the following information should the nurse include? (Select all that apply.)
   A. Use caffeine in moderation to prevent relapse.
   B. Difficulty sleeping can indicate a relapse.
   C. Begin taking your medications as soon as a relapse begins.
   D. Participating in psychotherapy can help prevent a relapse.
   E. Anhedonia is a clinical manifestation of a depressive relapse.

2. A nurse is assisting with planning care for a client who has bipolar disorder and is experiencing a manic episode. Sort the following items into interventions that the nurse should include or not include in the plan of care.
   A. Provide flexible client behavior expectations.
   B. Offer concise explanations.
   C. Establish consistent limits.
   D. Disregard client concerns.
   E. Use a firm approach with communication.

3. A nurse is discussing early indications of toxicity with a client who has a prescription for lithium carbonate for bipolar disorder. The nurse should include which of the following manifestations when reinforcing teaching? (Select all that apply.)
   A. Constipation
   B. Polyuria
   C. Rash
   D. Muscle weakness
   E. Tinnitus

4. A nurse is assisting with the admission of a client who has a new diagnosis of bipolar disorder and is scheduled to begin lithium therapy. When collecting a medical history from the client's caregiver, which of the following statements is the priority to report to the provider?
   A. "Current medical conditions include diabetes that is controlled by diet."
   B. "Recent medications include a course of prednisone for acute bronchitis."
   C. "Current vaccinations include a flu vaccine last month."
   D. "Current medications include furosemide for congestive heart failure."

5. A nurse is discussing routine follow-up needs with a client who has a prescription for valproate. The nurse should inform the client of the need for routine monitoring of which of the following?
   A. AST/ALT and LDH
   B. Creatinine and BUN
   C. WBC and granulocyte counts
   D. Blood sodium and potassium

Active Learning Scenario

A nurse in an acute mental health facility is assisting with the care of a client who is experiencing acute mania. Use the ATI Active Learning Template: System Disorder to complete this item, and include the following.

ALTERATIONS IN HEALTH (DIAGNOSIS)

EXPECTED FINDINGS: Identify four expected findings.

NURSING CARE: Identify two nursing actions.

CLIENT EDUCATION: Identify two client outcomes.

Active Learning Scenario Key

Using the ATI Active Learning Template: System Disorder

ALTERATIONS IN HEALTH (DIAGNOSIS): An abnormally elevated mood, which can also be described as expansive or irritable; usually requires hospitalization

EXPECTED FINDINGS
- Agitation and irritability
- Intolerance of interference or criticism
- Increase in talking and activity
- Flight of ideas
- Grandiosity
- Impulsivity
- Demanding and manipulative behavior
- Distractibility
- Poor judgment
- Attention-seeking behavior
- Impairment in social and occupational functioning
- Decreased sleep
- Neglect of ADLs
- Possible delusions and hallucinations
- Denial of illness

NURSING CARE
- Focus on safety as the priority of care.
- Maintain client's physical health and self-care needs.
- Assist with providing a safe environment.
- Monitor for suicidal thoughts, intentions, and escalating behavior.
- Decrease stimulation.
- Provide client protection with restraints, seclusion, or one-to-one observation if necessary.
- Implement frequent rest periods.
- Provide appropriate outlets for physical activity.
- Use calm and concise communication.

CLIENT EDUCATION: Client outcomes
- The client will refrain from self-harm.
- The client will sleep 6 to 8 hr each night.
- The client will maintain adequate fluid and food intake.
- The client will use appropriate communication skills to meet needs.
- The client will participate in self-care.

(N) *NCLEX® Connection: Psychosocial Integrity, Crisis Intervention*

Application Exercises Key

1. B, D, E. **CORRECT:** When taking action, the nurse should discuss relapse prevention with a client who has bipolar disorder and include the following information. The client should be alert for sleep disturbances, which can indicate a relapse. Also, the client who has bipolar disorder can participate in psychotherapy to help prevent a relapse. Additionally, the onset of anhedonia, the inability to feel pleasure, is a manifestation of depression, which can indicate a relapse of bipolar disorder. The client who has bipolar disorder should avoid the use of caffeine because it can precipitate a relapse. The client who has bipolar disorder should take prescribed medications to prevent and minimize a relapse.

   (N) *NCLEX® Connection: Psychosocial Integrity, Mental Health Concepts*

2. **INCLUDE:** B, C, E; **NOT INCLUDE:** A, D

   When assisting with planning care for the client who has bipolar disorder and is experiencing a manic episode, the nurse should include the following interventions in the plan of care. Offering concise explanations improves the client's ability to focus and comprehend the information. Establishing consistent limits decreases the risk for client manipulation. Using a firm approach with client communication promotes structure and minimizes inappropriate client behaviors. Establishing consistent client behavior expectations decreases the risk for client manipulation. Responding to valid client concerns fosters a trusting nurse-client relationship.

   (N) *NCLEX® Connection: Psychosocial Integrity, Behavioral Management*

3. B, D. **CORRECT:** When taking action, the nurse should discuss early indications of lithium carbonate for a client who has bipolar disorder, which include polyuria, muscle weakness, and diarrhea. A rash is not indication of lithium toxicity. Tinnitus is an indication of severe, rather than early, toxicity.

   (N) *NCLEX® Connection: Pharmacological Therapies, Adverse Effects/Contraindications/Adverse Effects/Interactions*

4. D. **CORRECT:** When collecting data from a client who is scheduled to begin lithium therapy, the nurse should recognize that it is priority to report to the provider the client's use of diuretics (furosemide) because they are contraindicated for use with lithium due to the risk for toxicity. This is the greatest risk for the client and is therefore the highest priority to report to the provider.

   (N) *NCLEX® Connection: Pharmacological Therapies, Adverse Effects/Contraindications/Adverse Effects/Interactions*

5. A. **CORRECT:** When taking action and discussing routine follow-up needs for a client who has a prescription for valproate, the nurse should inform the client that routine monitoring of liver function tests is necessary due to the risk for hepatotoxicity. Baseline levels can be drawn. However, routine monitoring of creatinine and BUN, WBC and granulocyte counts, and blood sodium and potassium are not necessary.

   (N) *NCLEX® Connection: Pharmacological Therapies, Adverse Effects/Contraindications/Side Effects/Interaction*

CHAPTER 15

CHAPTER 15 *Psychotic Disorders*

Schizophrenia spectrum and other psychotic disorders affect thinking, behavior, emotions, and the ability to perceive reality. Schizophrenia probably results from a combination of genetic, neurobiological, and nongenetic (injury at birth, viral infection, and nutritional) factors.

The typical age at onset is mid teens and mid 20s, but schizophrenia has occurred in young children and can begin in later adulthood. A prodromal period can occur during which the client experiences negative symptoms (anergia) or a reduced level of positive symptoms. Psychotic disorders become problematic when manifestations interfere with interpersonal relationships, self-care, and ability to work.

TYPES OF DISORDERS

The various types of psychotic disorders recognized and defined by the DSM-5-TR include the following.

Schizophrenia: The client has psychotic thinking or behavior present for at least 6 months. Areas of functioning, including school or work, self-care, and interpersonal relationships, are significantly impaired.

Schizotypal personality disorder: The client has impairments of personality (self and interpersonal) functioning. However, impairment is not as severe as with schizophrenia.

Delusional disorder: The client experiences delusional thinking for at least 1 month. Self or interpersonal functioning is not markedly impaired.

Brief psychotic disorder: The client has psychotic manifestations that last 1 day to 1 month in duration.

Schizophreniform disorder: The client has manifestations similar to schizophrenia, but the duration is 1 to 6 months, and social/occupational dysfunction might not be apparent.

Schizoaffective disorder: The client's disorder meets the criteria for both schizophrenia and depressive or bipolar disorder.

Substance/medication-induced psychotic disorder: The client experiences psychosis due to substance intoxication or withdrawal or after exposure to or withdrawal from a medication. However, the psychotic manifestations are more severe than typically expected.

Psychotic or catatonic disorder due to another medical condition: The client exhibits psychotic features (impaired reality testing), bizarre behavior (psychotic), or a significant change in motor activity behavior (catatonic), but does not meet criteria for diagnosis with another specific psychotic disorder.

DATA COLLECTION

EXPECTED FINDINGS

Characteristic dimensions of psychotic disorders

POSITIVE SYMPTOMS: Manifestation of things that are not normally present. These are the most easily identified manifestations.
- Hallucinations
- Delusions
- Alterations in speech
- Bizarre behavior (walking backward constantly)

NEGATIVE SYMPTOMS: Absence of things that are normally present. These manifestations are more difficult to treat successfully than positive symptoms.
- **Affect:** Usually blunted (narrow range of expression) or flat (facial expression never changes).
- **Alogia:** Poverty of thought or speech. The client might sit with a visitor but only mumble or respond vaguely to questions.
- **Anergia:** Lack of energy.
- **Anhedonia:** Lack of pleasure or joy. The client is indifferent to things that often make others happy, such as looking at beautiful scenery.
- **Avolition:** Lack of motivation in activities and hygiene. For example, the client completes an assigned task, such as making their bed, but is unable to start the next common chore without prompting.

COGNITIVE FINDINGS: Problems with thinking make it very difficult for the client to live independently.
- Disordered thinking
- Inability to make decisions
- Poor problem-solving ability
- Difficulty concentrating to perform tasks
- Short-term memory deficits
- Impaired abstract thinking

AFFECTIVE FINDINGS: Manifestations involving emotions
- Hopelessness
- Suicidal ideation
- Unstable or rapidly changing mood

Alterations in thought (delusions)

Alterations in thought are false fixed beliefs that cannot be corrected by reasoning and are usually bizarre. These include the following.
- **Ideas of reference:** Misconstrues trivial events and attaches personal significance to them, such as believing that others, who are discussing the next meal, are talking about them
- **Persecution:** Feels singled out for harm by others, such as being hunted down by the FBI

- **Grandeur:** Believes that they are all powerful and important, like a god
- **Somatic delusions:** Believes that their body is changing in an unusual way, such as growing a third arm
- **Jealousy:** Believes that their partner is sexually involved with another individual even though there is not any factual basis for this belief
- **Being controlled:** Believes that a force outside their body is controlling them
- **Thought broadcasting:** Believes that their thoughts are heard by others
- **Thought insertion:** Believes that others' thoughts are being inserted into their mind
- **Thought withdrawal:** Believes that their thoughts have been removed from their mind by an outside agency
- **Religiosity:** Is obsessed with religious beliefs
- **Magical thinking:** Believes their actions or thoughts are able to control a situation or affect others, such as wearing a certain hat makes them invisible to others

Alterations in speech

The following examples can occur.
- **Associative looseness:** Unconscious inability to concentrate on a single thought. Can progress to flight of ideas in which the client's speech moves so rapidly from one thought to another that it is incoherent
- **Neologisms:** Made-up words that have meaning only to the client ("I tranged and flittled.")
- **Echolalia:** The client repeats the words spoken to them.
- **Clang association:** Meaningless rhyming of words, often forceful, such as, "Oh fox, box, and lox."
- **Word salad:** Words jumbled together with little meaning or significance to the listener ("Hip hooray, the flip is cast and wide-sprinting in the forest.")
- **Circumstantiality:** Including multiple and unneeded details during a conversation, such as describing in great detail the weather and clothes they are wearing when asked what their plans are for the day
- **Tangentiality:** Starts talking about trivial information rather than focusing on the main topic of conversation, such as talking about what they will have for lunch when the discussion is about discharge medications

Alterations in perception

Hallucinations are sensory perceptions that do not have any apparent external stimulus. Examples include:
- **Auditory:** Hearing voices or sounds
  - **Command:** The voice instructs the client to perform an action (to hurt self or others). Qs
- **Visual:** Seeing persons or things
- **Olfactory:** Smelling odors
- **Gustatory:** Experiencing tastes
- **Tactile:** Feeling bodily sensations

Personal boundary difficulties

- Disenfranchisement with one's own body, identity, and perceptions. This includes the following.
  - **Depersonalization:** Nonspecific feeling that a client has lost their identity. Self is different or unreal
  - **Derealization:** Perception that the environment has changed, such as the client believing that objects in their environment are shrinking
  - **Illusions:** Misperceptions or misinterpretations of a real experience

Alterations in behavior

- **Extreme agitation:** Including pacing and rocking
- **Stereotyped behaviors:** Motor patterns that had meaning to client (sweeping the floor) but now are mechanical and lack purpose
- **Automatic obedience:** Responding in a robot-like manner
- **Waxy flexibility:** Maintaining a specific position for an extended period of time
- **Stupor:** Motionless for long periods of time, coma-like
- **Negativism:** Doing the opposite of what is requested
- **Echopraxia:** Purposeful imitation of movements made by others
- **Catatonia:** Pronounced decrease or increase in the amount of movement. Muscular rigidity, or catalepsy, may be so severe that limbs remain in whatever position they are placed.
- **Motor retardation:** Pronounced slowing of movement
- **Impaired impulse control:** Reduced ability to resist impulses
- **Gesturing or posturing:** Assuming unusual and illogical expressions
- **Boundary impairment:** Impaired ability to see where one person's body ends and another's begins

STANDARDIZED SCREENING TOOLS

Abnormal Involuntary Movement Scale (AIMS): This tool is used to monitor involuntary movements and tardive dyskinesia in clients who take antipsychotic medication. QEBP

PATIENT-CENTERED CARE

NURSING CARE

- Milieu therapy is used for clients who have a psychotic disorder both in acute mental health facilities and in community facilities (residential crisis centers, halfway houses, and day treatment programs).
  - Provide a structured, safe environment (milieu) for the client in order to decrease anxiety and to distract the client from constant thinking about hallucinations.
  - **Assertive Community Treatment (ACT):** Intensive case management and interprofessional team approach to assist clients with community-living needs. QTC

- Promote therapeutic communication to lower anxiety, decrease defensive patterns, and encourage participation in the milieu.
- Establish a trusting relationship with the client.
- Use appropriate communication to address hallucinations and delusions.
  - Ask the client directly about hallucinations. The nurse should not argue or agree with the client's view of the situation but can offer a comment, such as, "I don't hear anything, but you seem to be feeling frightened."
  - Do not argue with a client's delusions, but focus on the client's feelings and possibly offer reasonable explanations, such as, "I can't imagine that the president of the United States would have a reason to kill a citizen, but it must be frightening for you to believe that."
  - Monitor the client for paranoid delusions, which can increase the risk for violence against others.
  - If the client is experiencing command hallucinations, provide for safety due to the increased risk for harm to self or others. Qs
  - Attempt to focus conversations on reality-based subjects.
  - Identify manifestation triggers (loud noises [can trigger auditory hallucinations in certain clients]) and situations that seem to trigger conversations about the client's delusions.
  - Be genuine and empathetic in all dealings with the client.
- Determine discharge needs (ability to perform activities of daily living [ADLs]).
- Promote self-care by modeling and reinforcing teaching about self-care activities within the mental health facility.
- Relate wellness to the elements of manifestation management.
- Collaborate with the client to use manifestation management techniques to cope with depressive findings and anxiety. Manifestation management techniques include such strategies as using music to distract from "voices," attending activities, walking, talking to a trusted person when hallucinations are most bothersome, and interacting with an auditory or visual hallucination by telling it to stop or go away. Qpcc
- Reinforce teaching regarding medications.
- Whenever possible, incorporate family in all aspects of care.

CLIENT EDUCATION
- Develop social skills and friendships.
- Participate in group work and psychoeducation.
- Comply with the medication.

Medications for psychotic disorders

Schizophrenia spectrum disorders are the primary reason for the administration of antipsychotic medications. The clinical course of schizophrenia usually involves acute exacerbations with intervals of semi-remission in which manifestations remain present but are less severe.

Manifestations

Medications are used to treat the following.

POSITIVE SYMPTOMS RELATED TO BEHAVIOR, THOUGHT, PERCEPTION, AND SPEECH: Agitation, bizarre behavior, delusions, hallucinations, flight of ideas, loose associations

NEGATIVE SYMPTOMS: Social withdrawal, lack of emotion, lack of energy, flattened affect, decreased motivation, decreased pleasure in activities

GOALS OF TREATMENT

The goals of psychopharmacological treatment for schizophrenia and other psychotic disorders include the following.
- Suppression of acute episodes
- Prevention of acute recurrence
- Maintenance of the highest possible level of functioning

ANTIDEPRESSANTS

Used to treat the depression seen in many clients who have a psychotic disorder.

(Paroxetine)

NURSING ACTIONS
- Used temporarily to treat depression associated with psychotic disorders
- Monitor the client for suicidal ideation because this medication can increase thoughts of self-harm, especially when first taking it. Qs
- Notify the provider of any adverse effects (deepened depression).

CLIENT EDUCATION: Avoid abrupt cessation of this medication to avoid a withdrawal effect.

MOOD STABILIZING AGENTS AND BENZODIAZEPINES

Used to treat the anxiety often found in clients who have psychotic disorders, as well as some of the positive and negative symptoms.
- Valproate
- Lamotrigine
- Lorazepam

NURSING ACTIONS: Use these medications with caution in older adult clients.

CLIENT EDUCATION
- Medication could have sedative effects.
- Case management to provide follow-up for the client and family Qᴛᴄ
- Group, family, and individual psychoeducation to improve problem-solving and interpersonal skills
- Social skills training focuses on reinforcing teaching about social and ADL skills.

REINFORCE HEALTH TEACHING REGARDING THE FOLLOWING.
- Understanding of the disorder
- Need for self-care to prevent relapse
- Medication effects, adverse effects, and importance of compliance
- Importance of attending support groups
- Abstinence from the use of alcohol and/or other substances
- Keeping a log or journal of feelings and changes in behavior to help monitor medication effectiveness

FIRST-GENERATION ANTIPSYCHOTICS
- First-generation (conventional) antipsychotic medications are used mainly to control positive symptoms of psychotic disorders.
- Due to adverse effects, first-generation antipsychotic medications are reserved for clients who are:
  - Using them successfully and can tolerate the adverse effects
  - Concerned about the cost associated with second-generation antipsychotic medications
- First-generation agents are classified as either low, medium, or high potency depending on their association with extrapyramidal symptoms (EPSs), level of sedation, and anticholinergic adverse effects.
  - Low potency: low EPSs, high sedation, and high anticholinergic adverse effects
  - Medium potency: moderate EPSs, moderate sedation, and low anticholinergic adverse effects
  - High potency: high EPSs, low sedation, and low anticholinergic adverse effects

SECOND-GENERATION ANTIPSYCHOTICS
Second-generation (atypical) antipsychotic agents are often chosen as first-line treatment for schizophrenia. They are the current medications of choice for clients receiving initial treatment and for treating breakthrough episodes in clients on conventional medication therapy, because they are more effective with fewer adverse effects.

ADVANTAGES
- Relief of both positive and negative symptoms
- Decrease in affective findings (depression, anxiety) and suicidal behaviors
- Improvement of neurocognitive defects, such as poor memory
- Fewer or no EPSs, including tardive dyskinesia, due to less dopamine blockade

- Fewer anticholinergic effects, with the exception of clozapine, which has a high incidence of anticholinergic effects. This is because most of the atypical antipsychotics cause little or no blockade of cholinergic receptors.
- Less relapse

THIRD-GENERATION ANTIPSYCHOTICS
Third-generation antipsychotic agents are used to treat both positive and negative symptoms while improving cognitive function.

ADVANTAGES
- Decreased risk of EPSs or tardive dyskinesia
- Lower risk for weight gain and anticholinergic effects

Antipsychotics: first-generation (conventional)

SELECT PROTOTYPE MEDICATION: Chlorpromazine

OTHER MEDICATIONS
- Haloperidol, high potency
- Fluphenazine, high potency
- Loxapine, medium potency
- Thiothixene, high potency
- Perphenazine, medium potency

PURPOSE

EXPECTED PHARMACOLOGICAL ACTION
- First-generation antipsychotic medications block dopamine (D2), acetylcholine, histamine, and norepinephrine receptors in the brain and periphery.
- Inhibition of psychotic findings is believed to be a result of D2 blockade in the brain.

THERAPEUTIC USES
- Treatment of acute and chronic psychotic disorders
- Schizophrenia spectrum disorders
- Bipolar disorder: primarily the manic phase
- Tourette disorder
- Agitation
- Prevention of nausea/vomiting through blocking of dopamine in the chemoreceptor trigger zone of the medulla

COMPLICATIONS

Agranulocytosis

NURSING ACTIONS: If indications of infection appear, obtain a CBC. Medication should be discontinued if WBC count is less than 3,000 mm3.

CLIENT EDUCATION: Observe for indications of infection (fever, sore throat), and notify the provider if these occur.

Anticholinergic effects

MANIFESTATIONS

- Dry mouth
- Blurred vision
- Photophobia
- Urinary hesitancy or retention
- Constipation
- Tachycardia

NURSING ACTIONS: Suggest the following strategies to decrease anticholinergic effects.

- Chewing sugarless gum
- Sipping on water
- Avoiding hazardous activities
- Wearing sunglasses when outdoors
- Eating foods high in fiber
- Participating in regular exercise
- Maintaining fluid intake of 2 to 3 L/day from beverages and food sources
- Voiding just before taking medication

EXTRAPYRAMIDAL ADVERSE EFFECTS

Acute dystonia

MANIFESTATIONS

- Severe spasm of the tongue, neck, face, and back
- Crisis situation that requires rapid treatment

NURSING ACTIONS

- Begin to monitor for acute dystonia anywhere between 1 to 5 days after administration of first dose.
- Treat with an antiparkinsonian agents such as benztropine.
- IM or IV administration diphenhydramine can also be beneficial.
- Stay with the client and monitor the airway until spasms subside (usually 5 to 15 min).

Pseudoparkinsonism

MANIFESTATIONS

- Bradykinesia
- Positive symptoms of schizophrenia
- Rigidity
- Shuffling gait
- Drooling
- Tremors including pill-rolling
- Mask-like face

NURSING ACTIONS

- Observe for pseudoparkinsonism for the first month after the initiation of therapy. Can occur in 5 to 30 days following the first dose
- Treat with an antiparkinsonian agent (benztropine, trihexyphenidyl).
- Implement interventions to reduce the risk for falling.

Akathisia

MANIFESTATIONS

- Inability to sit or stand still
- Continual pacing and agitation

NURSING ACTIONS

- Observe for akathisia for the first 2 months after the initiation of treatment. Can occur in as little as 5 to 60 days following the first dose
- Manage with antiparkinsonian agents, beta blockers, or lorazepam/diazepam.
- Monitor for increased risk for suicide in clients who have severe akathisia.

Tardive dyskinesia (TD)

MANIFESTATIONS

- Late EPSs, which can require months to years of medication therapy for TD to develop
- Involuntary movements of the tongue and face, such as lip smacking and tongue fasciculations
- Involuntary movements of the arms, legs, and trunk

NURSING ACTIONS

- Evaluate the client after 12 months of therapy and then every 3 months. If TD appears, dosage should be lowered, or the client should be switched to a second-generation antipsychotic agent.
- Once TD develops, it usually does not decrease, even with discontinuation of the medication.
- There is no reliable treatment for TD.
- Reinforce to the client that purposeful muscle movement helps to control the involuntary TD.

Neuroendocrine effects

MANIFESTATIONS

- Gynecomastia
- Weight gain
- Menstrual irregularities
- Galactorrhea

NURSING ACTIONS: Monitor weight.

CLIENT EDUCATION: Observe for these manifestations and to notify the provider if they occur.

Neuroleptic malignant syndrome

MANIFESTATIONS

- Sudden high fever
- Blood pressure fluctuations
- Diaphoresis
- Tachycardia
- Muscle rigidity
- Decreased level of consciousness
- Coma

NURSING ACTIONS

- This life-threatening medical emergency can occur within the first week of treatment or any time thereafter.
- Stop antipsychotic medication.
- Monitor vital signs.
- Apply cooling blankets.
- Administer antipyretics.
- Increase the client's fluid intake.
- Administer dantrolene or bromocriptine to induce muscle relaxation.
- Administer medication as prescribed to treat arrhythmias.
- Assist with immediate transfer to an ICU.
- Wait 2 weeks before resuming therapy. Consider switching to an atypical agent.

Orthostatic hypotension

NURSING ACTIONS

- The client should develop tolerance in 2 to 3 months.
- Monitor blood pressure and heart rate for orthostatic changes. Hold medication until the provider is notified if there is a significant decrease in blood pressure or increase in heart rate.
- Encourage the client to increase fluid intake to maintain hydration.

CLIENT EDUCATION: If indications of orthostatic hypotension (lightheadedness, dizziness) occur, sit or lie down. Orthostatic hypotension can be minimized by getting up or changing positions slowly.

Sedation

CLIENT EDUCATION

- Effects should diminish within a few weeks.
- Take the medication at bedtime to avoid daytime sleepiness.
- Do not drive until sedation has subsided.

Seizures

INDICATIONS: Greatest risk in clients who have an existing seizure disorder

NURSING ACTIONS: An increase in antiseizure medication can be necessary.

CLIENT EDUCATION: Report seizure activity to the provider.

Severe dysrhythmias

NURSING ACTIONS

- Obtain baseline ECG and potassium level prior to treatment, and periodically throughout the treatment period.
- Avoid concurrent use with other medications that prolong QT interval.

Sexual dysfunction

Note: Common in all genders

NURSING ACTIONS: The client can need dosage lowered or be switched to a high-potency agent.

CLIENT EDUCATION

- Observe for possible adverse effects.
- Report effects to the provider.

Skin effects

MANIFESTATIONS

- Photosensitivity that can result in severe sunburn
- Contact dermatitis from handling medications

CLIENT EDUCATION

- Avoid excessive exposure to sunlight, use sunscreen, and wear protective clothing.
- Avoid direct contact with the medication.

Liver impairment

NURSING ACTIONS

- Monitor baseline liver function, and monitor periodically.
- Inform clients to observe for indications (anorexia, nausea, vomiting, fatigue, abdominal pain, jaundice) and to notify the provider.

CONTRAINDICATIONS/PRECAUTIONS

- These medications are contraindicated in clients who are in a coma or have Parkinson's disease, liver damage, or severe hypotension.
- Use of conventional antipsychotic medications is contraindicated in older adult clients who have dementia. Ⓖ
- Use cautiously in clients who have prostate enlargement, heart disorders, glaucoma, paralytic ileus, liver disease, kidney disease, or seizure disorders.

INTERACTIONS

Concurrent use with other anticholinergic medications increases effects.
CLIENT EDUCATION: Avoid over-the-counter medications that contain anticholinergic agents (sleep aids and antihistamines).

Additive CNS depressant effects with concurrent use of alcohol, opioids, and antihistamines

- CLIENT EDUCATION
  - Avoid alcohol and other medications that cause CNS depression.
  - Avoid hazardous activities, such as driving.

By activating dopamine receptors, levodopa counteracts effects of antipsychotic agents.
CLIENT EDUCATION: Avoid concurrent use of levodopa and other direct dopamine receptor agonists.

NURSING ADMINISTRATION

- Use the Abnormal Involuntary Movement Scale (AIMS) to screen for the presence of EPSs.
- Monitor the client to differentiate between EPSs and worsening of a psychotic disorder.
- Administer anticholinergics, beta blockers, and benzodiazepines to control early EPS. If adverse effects are intolerable, a client can be switched to a low-potency or atypical antipsychotic agent.
- Consider depot preparations (haloperidol decanoate, fluphenazine decanoate), administered IM once every 2 to 4 weeks, for clients who have difficulty maintaining a medication regimen. Inform the client that lower doses can be used with depot preparations, which will decrease the risk of adverse effects and the development of tardive dyskinesia. Ⓠpcc
- Begin administration with twice-daily dosing, but switch to daily dosing at bedtime to decrease daytime drowsiness and promote sleep.

CLIENT EDUCATION

- Antipsychotic medications rarely cause physical or psychological dependence.
- Take medication as prescribed and on a regular schedule.
- Some therapeutic effects can be noticeable within a few days, but significant improvement can take 2 to 4 weeks, and possibly several months for full effects.

Antipsychotics: second- and third-generation (atypical)

SELECT PROTOTYPE MEDICATION: Risperidone

OTHER MEDICATIONS
- Asenapine
- Clozapine
- Iloperidone
- Lurasidone
- Olanzapine
- Paliperidone
- Quetiapine
- Ziprasidone
- Aripiprazole (third generation)
- Cariprazine (third generation)
- Brexpiprazole (third generation)

PURPOSE

EXPECTED PHARMACOLOGICAL ACTION: These antipsychotic agents work mainly by blocking serotonin and, to a lesser degree, dopamine receptors. These medications also block receptors for norepinephrine, histamine, and acetylcholine. The third-generation medications work by stabilizing the dopamine system as both an agonist and antagonist.

THERAPEUTIC USES
- Negative and positive symptoms of schizophrenia spectrum disorders
- Psychosis induced by levodopa therapy
- Relief of psychotic manifestations in other disorders, such as bipolar disorder
- Impulse control disorders

COMPLICATIONS

Agranulocytosis

NURSING ACTIONS
- Advise clients to observe for indications of infection.
- If indications of infection appear, obtain a CBC.
- Onset is gradual and usually occurs during the first 6 months of therapy.
- Can occur with chlorpromazine

Metabolic syndrome

- New onset of diabetes mellitus or loss of glucose control in clients who have diabetes
- Dyslipidemia with increased risk for hypertension and other cardiovascular disease
- Weight gain

NURSING ACTIONS
- Obtain baseline fasting blood glucose, and monitor the value periodically throughout treatment.
- Monitor cholesterol, triglycerides, and blood glucose if weight gain is greater than 14 kg (31 lb).

CLIENT EDUCATION
- Report indications (increased thirst, urination, appetite) to the provider.
- Follow a healthy, low-calorie diet, engage in regular exercise, and monitor weight gain.

Orthostatic hypotension

NURSING ACTIONS
- Monitor blood pressure and heart rate for orthostatic changes.
- Hold medication while notifying the provider of significant changes.

Anticholinergic effects

Such as urinary hesitancy or retention, dry mouth

NURSING ACTIONS
- Monitor for these adverse effects, and report their occurrence to the provider.
- Encourage the client to use measures to relieve dry mouth, such as sipping water throughout the day.

Agitation, dizziness, sedation, sleep disruption

NURSING ACTIONS
- Monitor for these adverse effects, and report their occurrence to the provider.
- Administer an alternative medication if prescribed.

Mild EPS, such as tremor

NURSING ACTIONS
- Monitor for and instruct clients to recognize EPS.
- Use AIMS test to screen for EPS.

Elevated prolactin levels

NURSING ACTIONS: Obtain prolactin level if indicated.

CLIENT EDUCATION: Observe for galactorrhea, gynecomastia, and amenorrhea, and notify the provider if these occur.

Sexual dysfunction

Anorgasmia, impotence, low libido

CLIENT EDUCATION
- Observe for possible sexual adverse effects.
- Notify provider if intolerable.
- Methods for managing sexual dysfunction can include using adjunct medications to improve sexual function, such as sildenafil.

CONTRAINDICATIONS/PRECAUTIONS

Risperidone

- These medications should not be used for clients who have dementia. Use of these medications can cause death related to cerebrovascular accident or infection. Qs
- Clients should avoid the concurrent use of alcohol.
- Use cautiously in clients who have cardiovascular or cerebrovascular disease, seizures, or diabetes mellitus. Clients who have diabetes mellitus should have a baseline fasting blood sugar, and blood glucose should be monitored carefully.

OTHER ATYPICAL ANTIPSYCHOTIC AGENTS

Aripiprazole (third-generation antipsychotic)

- Tablets
- Orally disintegrating tablets
- Oral solution
- Short-acting injectable
- Long-acting injectable

NURSING ACTIONS
- Low or no risk of EPS
- Low or no risk of diabetes, weight gain, dyslipidemia, orthostatic hypotension, and anticholinergic effects

ADVERSE EFFECTS
- Sedation
- Headache
- Anxiety
- Insomnia
- Gastrointestinal upset

Asenapine

Sublingual tablets

NURSING ACTIONS: Low risk of diabetes, weight gain, dyslipidemia, and anticholinergic effects. Warn clients not to swallow tablets, and instruct to avoid eating and drinking for 10 minutes after dosing.

OTHER ADVERSE EFFECTS
- Drowsiness
- Prolonged QT interval
- EPS (higher doses)
- Causes temporary numbing of the mouth

Clozapine

The first atypical antipsychotic developed, it is no longer considered a first-line medication for schizophrenia spectrum disorders due to its adverse effects.
- Tablets
- Orally disintegrating tablets

NURSING ACTIONS
- Low risk of EPS
- High risk of weight gain, diabetes, and dyslipidemia
- Risk for fatal agranulocytosis, typically occurs within the first 6 months with gradual onset

- Baseline and regular monitoring of WBC per protocol (weekly, bi-weekly, then monthly) required
- Notification of the provider of indications of infection (fever, sore throat, mouth lesions) is necessary.

OTHER ADVERSE EFFECTS
- Sedation
- Orthostatic hypotension
- Hypersalivation
- Anticholinergic effects

Iloperidone

Tablets

NURSING ACTIONS
- Significant risk for weight gain, prolonged QT interval, and orthostatic hypotension
- Low risk for diabetes, dyslipidemia, and EPS

CLIENT EDUCATION: Follow titration schedule during initial therapy to minimize hypotension.

COMMON ADVERSE EFFECTS
- Dry mouth
- Sedation
- Fatigue
- Nasal congestion

Lurasidone

Tablets

NURSING ACTIONS
- Low risk for diabetes, weight gain, and dyslipidemia
- Does not cause anticholinergic effects
- Administer with food, at least 350 kcals, for maximum absorption.

COMMON ADVERSE EFFECTS
- Sedation
- Akathisia
- Parkinsonism
- Agitation and anxiety
- Nausea

Olanzapine

- Orally disintegrating tablets
- Short-acting injectable
- Extended-release injection

NURSING ACTIONS
- Low risk of EPS
- High risk of diabetes, weight gain, and dyslipidemia

OTHER ADVERSE EFFECTS
- Sedation
- Orthostatic hypotension
- Anticholinergic effects

! Following administration of extended-release injection, the client requires observation for at least 3 hr to monitor for adverse effects.

Paliperidone

- Extended-release tablets
- Extended-release injections

NURSING ACTIONS: Significant risk for diabetes, weight gain, and dyslipidemia

OTHER ADVERSE EFFECTS
- Sedation
- Prolonged QT interval
- Orthostatic hypotension
- Anticholinergic effects
- Mild EPS

Quetiapine

- Tablets
- Extended-release tablets

NURSING ACTIONS
- Low risk of EPS
- Moderate risk of diabetes, weight gain, and dyslipidemia

OTHER ADVERSE EFFECTS
- Cataracts
- Sedation
- Orthostatic hypotension
- Anticholinergic effects

Ziprasidone

This medication affects both dopamine and serotonin, so it can be used for clients who have concurrent depression.
- Capsules
- Short-acting injectable

NURSING ACTIONS
- Low risk of EPS
- Low risk of diabetes, weight gain, and dyslipidemia
- For maximum absorption, administer with food.

OTHER ADVERSE EFFECTS
- Sedation
- Orthostatic hypotension
- Anticholinergic effects
- ECG changes and QT prolongation that can lead to torsades de pointes

INTERACTIONS

Immunosuppressive medications, such as anticancer medications, can further suppress immune function.
NURSING ACTIONS: Avoid use in clients who are taking clozapine.

Additive CNS depressant effects can occur with concurrent use of alcohol, opioids, antihistamines, and other CNS depressants.
- CLIENT EDUCATION
  - Avoid alcohol and other medications that cause CNS depression.
  - Avoid hazardous activities, such as driving.

By activating dopamine receptors, levodopa counteracts the effects of antipsychotic agents.
NURSING ACTIONS: Avoid concurrent use of levodopa and other direct dopamine receptor agonists.

Tricyclic antidepressants, amiodarone, and clarithromycin prolong QT intervals, thereby increasing the risk of cardiac dysrhythmias.
NURSING ACTIONS: Atypical antipsychotics that prolong the QT interval should not be used concurrently with other medications that have the same effect.

Barbiturates and phenytoin stimulate hepatic medication-metabolizing enzymes, thereby decreasing medication levels of aripiprazole, quetiapine, and ziprasidone.
NURSING ACTIONS: Monitor medication effectiveness.

Fluconazole inhibits hepatic medication-metabolizing enzymes, thereby increasing medication levels of aripiprazole, quetiapine, and ziprasidone.
NURSING ACTIONS: Monitor medication effectiveness.

NURSING ADMINISTRATION

Risperidone also is available as a depot injection administered IM once every 2 weeks, and the extended-release injection of paliperidone is administered every 28 days. LAI Invega Trinza is administered every 3 months (paliperidone palmitate: generic). Aripiprazole also has a long-acting injectable, which is administered on a monthly basis. This method of administration is a good option for clients who have difficulty adhering to a medication schedule. Therapeutic effect occurs 2 to 6 weeks after first depot injection.
- Use oral disintegrating tablets for clients who can attempt to "cheek" or "pocket" tablets or for those who have difficulty swallowing them.
- Administer lurasidone and ziprasidone with food to increase absorption.
- The cost of antipsychotic medications can be a factor for some clients. Monitor the need for case management intervention. Qᴛᴄ

CLIENT EDUCATION
- Low doses of medication are given initially, and dosages are then gradually increased. ("Start low and go slow.")
- If taking asenapine, avoid eating or drinking for 10 min after each dose.

NURSING EVALUATION OF MEDICATION EFFECTIVENESS

Depending on therapeutic intent, effectiveness can be evidenced by the following.
- Improvement and/or prevention of acute psychotic manifestations, absence of hallucinations, delusions, anxiety, hostility
- Improvement in ability to perform ADLs
- Improvement in ability to interact socially with peers
- Improvement of sleeping and eating habits

Application Exercises

1. Determine which symptoms are is positive or negative symptoms of schizophrenia.
   A. Hallucinations
   B. Avolition
   C. Alterations in speech
   D. Delusions
   E. Bizarre motor movements
   F. Flat affect
   G. Anhedonia
   H. Anergia

2. A nurse is speaking with a client who has schizophrenia when the client suddenly seems to stop focusing on the nurse's questions and begins looking at the ceiling and talking to themselves. Which of the following actions should the nurse take?
   A. Stop the interview at this point, and resume later when the client is better able to concentrate.
   B. Ask the client, "Are you seeing something on the ceiling?"
   C. Tell the client, "You seem to be looking at something on the ceiling. I see something there, too."
   D. Continue the interview without commenting on the client's behavior.

3. A nurse is discussing manifestations of schizophrenia with a newly licensed nurse. Which of the following manifestations should the nurse identify as being effectively treated by first-generation antipsychotics? (Select all that apply.)
   A. Auditory hallucinations
   B. Withdrawal from social situations
   C. Delusions of grandeur
   D. Severe agitation
   E. Anhedonia

4. A nurse is caring for a client who is currently taking perphenazine. Which of the following findings should the nurse identify as an extrapyramidal symptom (EPS)? (Select all that apply.)
   A. Decreased level of consciousness
   B. Drooling
   C. Involuntary arm movements
   D. Urinary retention
   E. Continual pacing

5. Determine which category each medication listed below belongs to: typical antipsychotics or atypical antipsychotics.
   A. Risperidone
   B. Haloperidol
   C. Quetiapine
   D. Loxapine
   E. Olanzapine
   F. Clozapine

Active Learning Scenario

A nurse is caring for a client who has schizophrenia and is reviewing discharge instructions, which include a new prescription for risperidone. Use the ATI Active Learning Template: Medication to complete the following.

THERAPEUTIC USE: Identify the therapeutic uses of risperidone.

CLIENT EDUCATION: Describe at least three education points.

Application Exercises Key

1. **POSITIVE:** A, C, D, E; **NEGATIVE:** B, F, G, H

   Some examples of positive symptoms of schizophrenia include hallucinations, alterations in speech, delusions, and bizarre motor movements. Examples of negative symptoms of schizophrenia include avolition, anhedonia, anergia, and flat affect.

   Ⓝ *NCLEX® Connection: Psychosocial Integrity, Mental Health Concepts*

2. B. **CORRECT:** When taking action, the nurse should ask the client directly about the hallucination to identify client needs and monitor for a potential risk for injury. The nurse should address the client's current needs related to the possible hallucination rather than to stop the interview. Also, avoid agreeing with the client, which can promote psychotic thinking. The nurse should address the client's current needs related to the possible hallucinations rather than ignoring the change in behavior.

   Ⓝ *NCLEX® Connection: Psychosocial Integrity, Mental Health Concepts*

3. A, C, D. **CORRECT:** When taking action, the nurse should identify that auditory hallucinations, delusions of grandeur, and severe agitation are positive symptoms of schizophrenia that are effectively treated by first-generation antipsychotics. First-generation antipsychotics have minimal effectiveness with negative symptoms of schizophrenia such as anhedonia and withdrawal from social situations.

   Ⓝ *NCLEX® Connection: Pharmacological Therapies, Expected Actions/Outcomes*

4. B, C, E. **CORRECT:** When collecting data for a client, the nurse should identify that drooling is an indication of pseudoparkinsonism, which is an EPS. Involuntary arm movements are an indication of tardive dyskinesia, which is an EPS. Continual pacing is an indication of akathisia, which is an EPS. Urinary retention is an anticholinergic effect rather than an EPS. Decreased level of consciousness is an indication of neuroleptic malignant syndrome rather than an EPS.

   Ⓝ *NCLEX® Connection: Pharmacological Therapies, Adverse Effects/Contraindications/Adverse Effects/Interactions*

5. **TYPICAL ANTIPSYCHOTICS:** B, D;
   ATYPICAL ANTIPSYCHOTICS: A, C, E, F

   The nurse should determine that atypical antipsychotics are risperidone, quetiapine, olanzapine, and clozapine. Typical antipsychotics are haloperidol and loxapine.

   Ⓝ *NCLEX® Connection: Pharmacological Therapies, Expected Actions/Outcomes*

Active Learning Scenario Key

Using the ATI Active Learning Template: Medication

THERAPEUTIC USE: Risperidone is a second-generation/atypical antipsychotic medication used to treat positive and negative symptoms of schizophrenia.

CLIENT EDUCATION
- Advise the client to follow a balanced diet.
- Recommend regular exercise.
- Instruct the client to monitor weight.
- Reinforce teaching about adverse effects (agitation, dizziness, sedation, sleep disruption) and instruct the client to notify their provider if they are present.

Ⓝ *NCLEX® Connection: Pharmacological Therapies, Adverse Effects/Contraindications/Adverse Effects/Interactions*

UNIT 3 PSYCHOBIOLOGIC DISORDERS

CHAPTER 16 *Personality Disorders*

A client who has a personality disorder demonstrates pathological personality characteristics, including impairments in self-identity/self-direction and interpersonal functioning.

The maladaptive behaviors of a personality disorder are not always perceived by the individual as dysfunctional, and some areas of personal functioning can be adequate.

Personality disorders often co-occur with other mental health diagnoses (depression, anxiety, and eating and substance use disorders).

DATA COLLECTION

RISK FACTORS

- Clients who have personality disorders often have comorbid substance use disorders and can have a history of nonviolent and violent crimes, including sex offenses.
- Psychosocial influences (childhood abuse or trauma) and developmental factors with a direct link to parenting
- Biological influences include genetic and biochemical factors.

EXPECTED FINDINGS

Clients who have a personality disorder exhibit one or more of the following common pathological personality characteristics.

- Inflexibility/maladaptive responses to stress
- Compulsiveness and lack of social restraint
- Inability to emotionally connect in social and professional relationships
- Tendency to provoke interpersonal conflict

DEFENSE MECHANISMS

Defense mechanisms used by clients who have personality disorders include repression, suppression, regression, undoing, and splitting.

- Of these, splitting, which is the inability to incorporate positive and negative aspects of oneself or others into a whole image, is frequently seen in the acute mental health setting. Q EBP
- Splitting is commonly associated with borderline personality disorder.
- In splitting, the client tends to characterize people or things as all good or all bad at any particular moment. For example, the client might say, "You are the worst person in the world." Later that day, they might say, "You are the best, but the nurse from the last shift is absolutely terrible."

LIFESPAN CONSIDERATIONS

- Children may exhibit difficulties in developing social relationships and school classwork.
- Adolescents may report being bullied for having odd habits, behaviors, or ideas.
- Adults may have trouble forming intimate relationships, maintaining or establishing careers, and fulfilling opportunities to mentor future generations.

16.1 Case study

Scenario Introduction

A nurse is discussing with a newly licensed nurse the characteristics of personality disorders.

Scene 1

Nurse Russell: "It is important, Quinn, that you have an understanding of the various characteristics of personality disorders. Tell me more about characteristics each personality disorder has."

Newly Licensed Nurse Quinn: "Russell, I need to take a minute to think of them. I am going to write down the clinical findings for each disorder."

Scenario conclusion

The newly licensed nurse begins to group clinical findings with the associated personality disorder.

Case study exercises

1. Sort the following characteristics to the appropriate personality disorder: Antisocial, Borderline, or Narcissistic.
   A. Sense of entitlement
   B. Instability of affect
   C. Splitting behaviors
   D. Fear of abandonment
   E. Arrogance
   F. Need for consistent admiration

2. As a newly licensed nurse, what interventions should the nurse include in the plan of care for a client who has concerns regarding safety?

THE 10 PERSONALITY DISORDERS

Cluster A (odd or eccentric traits)

- **Paranoid:** Characterized by distrust and suspiciousness toward others based on unfounded beliefs that others want to harm, exploit, or deceive the person
- **Schizoid:** Characterized by emotional detachment, disinterest in close relationships, and indifference to praise or criticism; often uncooperative
- **Schizotypal:** Characterized by odd beliefs leading to interpersonal difficulties, an eccentric appearance, and magical thinking or perceptual distortions that are not clear delusions or hallucinations

Cluster B (dramatic, emotional, or erratic traits)

- **Antisocial:** Characterized by disregard for others with exploitation, lack of empathy, repeated unlawful actions, deceit, failure to accept personal responsibility; evidence of conduct disorder before age 15, sense of entitlement, manipulative, impulsive, and seductive behaviors; nonadherence to traditional morals and values; verbally charming and engaging
- **Borderline:** Characterized by instability of affect, identity, and relationships, as well as splitting behaviors, manipulation, impulsiveness, and fear of abandonment; often self-injurious and potentially suicidal; ideas of reference are common; often accompanied by impulsivity
- **Histrionic:** Characterized by emotional attention-seeking behavior, in which the person needs to be the center of attention; often seductive and flirtatious
- **Narcissistic:** Characterized by arrogance, grandiose views of self-importance, the need for consistent admiration, and a lack of empathy for others that strains most relationships; often sensitive to criticism

Cluster C (anxious or fearful traits; insecurity and inadequacy)

- **Avoidant:** Characterized by social inhibition and avoidance of all situations that require interpersonal contact, despite wanting close relationships, due to extreme fear of rejection; have feelings of inadequacy and are anxious in social situations
- **Dependent:** Characterized by extreme dependency in a close relationship with an urgent search to find a replacement when one relationship ends
- **Obsessive-compulsive:** Characterized by indecisiveness and perfectionism with a focus on orderliness and control to the extent that the individual might not be able to accomplish a given task

PATIENT-CENTERED CARE

NURSING CARE

- Self-assessment is vital for nurses caring for clients who have personality disorders and should be performed prior to care.
  - Clients who have personality disorders can evoke intense emotions in the nurse.
  - Awareness of personal reactions to stress promotes effective nursing care.
  - Therapeutic communication and intervention are promoted when client behaviors are anticipated.
  - The nurse should repeat the self-assessment if experiencing a personal stress response to client behavior.
- Milieu management focuses on appropriate social interaction within a group context.
- Safety is always a priority concern because some clients who have a personality disorder are at risk for self-injury or violence. Qs
  - Clients diagnosed with borderline personality disorder are at a higher risk for danger to self.
  - Clients diagnosed with anti-social personality disorder are at a higher risk for danger to others.
- The plan of care for clients who have personality disorders varies according to the cluster they are in.
  - **Cluster A:** Emphasize client skill and resource development in finding and maintaining interpersonal relationships.
  - **Cluster B:** Develop skills to limit dramatic and inappropriate behaviors.
  - **Cluster C:** Reinforce education and therapies to learn how to best manage feelings of anxiety.

COMMUNICATION STRATEGIES

Developing a therapeutic relationship is often challenging due to the client's distrust or hostility toward others. Feelings of being threatened or having no control can cause a client to act out toward the nurse.

- A firm, yet supportive approach and consistent care will help build a therapeutic nurse-client relationship.
- Offer the client realistic choices to enhance the client's sense of control.
- Limit-setting and consistency are essential with clients who are manipulative, especially those who have borderline or antisocial personality disorders. QEBP
- Clients who have dependent and histrionic personality disorders often benefit from assertiveness training and modeling as well as psychotherapy.
- Clients who have schizoid or schizotypal personality disorders tend to isolate themselves, and the nurse should respect this need. Psychotherapy can help improve the client's ability to respond to social cues from others.
- For clients who have histrionic personality disorder and can be flirtatious, it is important for the nurse to maintain professional boundaries and communication at all times.
- When caring for clients who exhibit dependent behavior, self-assess frequently for countertransference reactions.

MEDICATIONS

Medications include the use of psychotropic agents to provide relief from manifestations. Antidepressant, anxiolytic, antipsychotic, or mood stabilizer medications may be prescribed.

INTERPROFESSIONAL CARE

Psychobiological interventions

- Psychotherapy, group therapy, and cognitive and behavior therapy are effective treatment modalities for clients who have personality disorders.
- Dialectical behavior therapy is a cognitive-behavioral therapy used for clients who exhibit self-injurious behavior. It focuses on gradual behavior changes and provides acceptance and validation for these clients.
- Case management is beneficial for clients who have personality disorders and are persistently and severely impaired.
  - In acute care facilities, case management focuses on obtaining pertinent history from current or previous providers, supporting reintegration with the family, and ensuring appropriate referrals to outpatient care.
  - In long-term outpatient facilities, case management goals include reducing hospitalization by providing resources for crisis services and enhancing the social support system. Qᴛᴄ

Active Learning Scenario

A nurse is discussing self-assessment with a newly licensed nurse. Use the ATI Active Learning Template: Basic Concept to complete this item.

RELATED CONTENT: Identify how self-assessment relates to caring for a client who has a personality disorder.

UNDERLYING PRINCIPLES: Identify at least two concepts.

NURSING INTERVENTIONS: Identify who should perform self-assessment and when it is indicated.

Active Learning Scenario Key

Using the ATI Active Learning Template: Basic Concept

RELATED CONTENT: Self-assessment is vital for nurses caring for clients who have personality disorders because of the intense emotions that can be elicited during client care.

UNDERLYING PRINCIPLES
- Self-assessment prepares the nurse for the personal emotions that can be experienced as a result of client care.
- The nurse can provide more effective nursing care when aware of personal reactions to stress.
- Therapeutic communication and intervention are promoted when client behaviors are anticipated.

NURSING INTERVENTIONS
- **Who:** Self-assessment should be performed by all nurses caring for a client who has a personality disorder.
- **When:** Perform a self-assessment prior to providing client care and whenever experiencing a personal stress response to client behavior.

Ⓝ *NCLEX® Connection: Psychosocial Integrity, Stress Management*

1. A nurse is caring for a client who has borderline personality disorder. The client says, "The nurse on the evening shift is always nice! You are the meanest nurse ever!" The nurse should recognize the client's statement as an example of which of the following defense mechanisms?
   - A. Regression
   - B. Splitting
   - C. Undoing
   - D. Identification

2. A nurse is caring for a client who has avoidant personality disorder. Which of the following statements is expected from a client who has this type of personality disorder?
   - A. "I'm scared that you're going to leave me."
   - B. "I'll go to group therapy if you'll let me smoke."
   - C. "I need to feel that everyone admires me."
   - D. "I sometimes feel better if I cut myself."

3. A nurse is assisting with a court-ordered evaluation of a client who has antisocial personality disorder. Which of the following findings should the nurse expect? (Select all that apply.)
   - A. Demonstrates extreme anxiety when placed in a social situation
   - B. Often engages in magical thinking
   - C. Attempts to convince other clients to relinquish their belongings
   - D. Becomes agitated if personal area is not neat and orderly
   - E. Blames others for personal past and current problems

4. A nurse is assisting with the preparation of a staff education session on personality disorders. Which of the following personality characteristics associated with all of the personality disorders should the nurse include? (Select all that apply.)
   - A. Difficulty in getting along with other members of a group
   - B. Belief in the ability to become invisible during times of stress
   - C. Display of defense mechanisms when routines are changed
   - D. Claiming to be more important than other persons
   - E. Difficulty understanding why it is inappropriate to have a personal relationship with staff

5. A nurse is discussing the care of a client who has a personality disorder with a newly licensed nurse. Which of the following statements by the newly licensed nurse indicates an understanding of the discussion?
   - A. "I can promote my client's sense of control by establishing a schedule."
   - B. "I should encourage clients who have a schizoid personality disorder to increase socialization."
   - C. "I should practice limit-setting to help prevent client manipulation."
   - D. "I should implement assertiveness training with clients who have antisocial personality disorder."

Application Exercises Key

1. B. **CORRECT:** Splitting occurs when a person is unable to see both positive and negative qualities at the same time. The client who has borderline personality disorder tends to see a person as all bad one time and all good another time. Regression refers to resorting to an earlier way of functioning (having a temper tantrum). Undoing is a behavior that is intended to undo or reverse unacceptable thoughts or acts (buying a gift for a spouse after having an extramarital affair). In identification, the person imitates the behavior of someone admired or feared.

   Ⓝ *NCLEX® Connection: Psychosocial Integrity, Mental Health Concepts*

2. A. **CORRECT:** Clients who have avoidant personality disorder often have a fear of abandonment. This type of statement is expected.
   B. This statement indicates manipulation, which is expected from a client who has antisocial personality disorder.
   C. This statement indicates a need for admiration, which is expected from a client who has narcissistic personality disorder.
   D. This statement indicates a risk for self-injury, which is expected from a client who has borderline personality disorder.

   Ⓝ *NCLEX® Connection: Psychosocial Integrity, Mental Health Concepts*

3. C, E. **CORRECT:** Exploitation and manipulation of others is an expected finding of antisocial personality disorder. Failure to accept personal responsibility is an expected finding of clients who have antisocial personality disorder. Anxiety in social situations is an expected finding of clients who have avoidant personality disorder. Magical thinking and odd beliefs are findings observed in clients who have schizotypal personality disorder. Perfectionism with a focus on orderliness and control is an expected finding of clients who have obsessive-compulsive personality disorder.

   Ⓝ *NCLEX® Connection: Psychosocial Integrity, Mental Health Concepts*

4. A, C, E. **CORRECT:** Difficulty with social and professional relationships is a personality characteristic that can be seen with all personality disorder types. Maladaptive response to stress is a personality characteristic that can be seen in clients who are experiencing personality disorders. Difficulty understanding personal boundaries is a personality characteristic that can be seen with all personality disorder types. Clients who have schizotypal personality disorder can display magical thinking or delusions. However, this is not associated with all personality disorder types. Clients who have narcissistic personality disorder can display grandiose thinking. However, this is not associated with all personality disorder types.

   Ⓝ *NCLEX® Connection: Psychosocial Integrity, Mental Health Concepts*

5. C. **CORRECT:** When caring for a client who has a personality disorder, limit-setting is appropriate to help prevent client manipulation. Rather than establishing a schedule, the nurse should ask for the client's input and offer realistic choices to promote the client's sense of control. Avoid trying to increase socialization for a client who has a schizoid personality disorder. Implement assertiveness training for clients who have dependent and histrionic personality disorders.

   Ⓝ *NCLEX® Connection: Psychosocial Integrity, Mental Health Concepts*

Case Study Exercises Key

1. **ANTISOCIAL:** A; **BORDERLINE:** B, C, D; **NARCISSISTIC:** E, F

   Clients who have borderline personality disorder exhibit instability of affect, splitting behaviors, and fear of abandonment.

   Ⓝ *NCLEX® Connection: Psychosocial Integrity, Mental Health Concepts*

2. Safety is always a priority concern because some clients who have a personality disorder are at risk for self-injury or violence. Clients diagnosed with borderline personality disorder are at a higher risk for danger to self. Clients diagnosed with anti-social personality disorder are at a higher risk for danger to others.

   Ⓝ *NCLEX® Connection: Safety and Infection Control, Accident/Error/Injury Prevention*

CHAPTER 17 Neurocognitive Disorders

Neurocognitive disorders are a group of conditions characterized by the disruption of thinking, memory, processing, and problem-solving. Treatment of clients who have neurocognitive disorders requires a compassionate understanding of both the client and family.

TYPES OF COGNITIVE DISORDERS

- Cognitive disorders recognized and defined by the DSM-5 -TR include the following.
  - **Delirium**
  - **Mild neurocognitive disorder (NCD)**
  - **Major neurocognitive disorder** (commonly known as **dementia**)
- Although delirium tends to be short-term and reversible, mild neurocognitive disorders may or may not progress to a major disorder. Major disorders are progressive and irreversible.
- Major and mild NCD subtypes are further classified (NCD due to Alzheimer's disease, NCD due to Parkinson's disease, or NCD due to Huntington's disease).
  - **Alzheimer's disease (AD)** is a subtype of NCD that is neurodegenerative, resulting in the gradual impairment of cognitive function. It is the most common type of major NCD.
- It is important to distinguish between a cognitive disorder and other mental health disorders that can have similar manifestations. Depression in the older adult can mimic the early stages of Alzheimer's disease. ⓖ

DATA COLLECTION

RISK FACTORS

- Risk factors for delirium include physiological changes, including neurologic (Parkinson's disease, Huntington's disease), metabolic (hepatic or kidney failure, fluid and electrolyte imbalances, nutritional deficiencies), cardiovascular and respiratory diseases, infections (HIV/AIDS), surgery, and substance use or withdrawal.
- Other risk factors for delirium include older age, multiple comorbidities, severity of disease, polypharmacy, intensive care units, surgery, aphasia, restraint use, and change in client environment.
- Risk factors for neurocognitive disorder and AD include advanced age, prior head trauma, cardiovascular disease, lifestyle factors, and a family history of AD. There is a strong genetic link in early-onset familial AD.

EXPECTED FINDINGS

- Delirium and neurocognitive disorder have some similarities and some important differences. (17.1)
- Clients who have NCD can also develop delirium.

DEFENSE MECHANISMS

Clients often use defense mechanisms to preserve self-esteem and to compensate when cognitive changes are progressive.

Denial: Both the client and family members can refuse to believe that changes (loss of memory) are taking place, even when those changes are obvious to others.

Confabulation: The client can make up stories when questioned about events or activities that they do not remember. This can seem like lying, but it is actually an unconscious attempt to save self-esteem and prevent admitting the inability to remember the occasion.

Perseveration: The client avoids answering questions by repeating phrases or behavior. This is another unconscious attempt to maintain self-esteem when memory has failed.

DIAGNOSTIC PROCEDURES ⓠEBP

There is no specific laboratory or diagnostic testing to diagnose NCDs. Definitive diagnosis cannot be made until autopsy. Testing is done to rule out other pathologies that could be mistaken for NCDs.

- Chest and head x-rays
- Electroencephalography (EEG)
- Electrocardiography (ECG)
- Liver function studies
- Thyroid function tests
- Neuroimaging (computer tomography and positron emission tomography of the brain)
- Urinalysis
- Blood electrolytes
- Folate and vitamin B_{12} levels
- Vision and hearing tests
- Lumbar puncture

SCREENING/DATA COLLECTION TOOLS

Confusion Assessment Method (CAM): For delirium

Neelon-Champagne (NEECHAM) Confusion Scale: For delirium

Functional Dementia Scale: This tool will give the nurse information regarding the client's ability to perform self-care, extent of the client's memory loss, mood changes, and the degree of danger to self and/or others. ⓠEBP

Mini-mental status examination (MMSE)

Functional Assessment Screening Tool (FAST)

Global Deterioration Scale

Short Blessed Test: This tool provides the nurse with client behavioral information based on an interview with a secondary source (a client's family member).

PATIENT-CENTERED CARE

NURSING CARE

- The best way to prevent and manage delirium is to minimize risk factors and promote early detection. Timely recognition is essential.
- Perform self-assessment regarding possible feelings of frustration, anger, or fear when performing daily care for clients who have progressive cognitive decline.
- Nursing interventions are focused on protecting the client from injury, as well as promoting client dignity and quality of life.
- Provide for a safe and therapeutic environment. Qs
  - Collect data for potential injury, such as falls or wandering.
  - Assign the client to a room close to the nurses' station for close observation.
  - Provide a room with a low level of visual and auditory stimuli.
  - Provide for a well-lit environment, minimizing contrasts and shadows.
  - Have the client sit in a room with windows to help with time orientation.
  - Have the client wear an identification bracelet. Use monitors and bed alarm devices as needed.
  - Use restraints only as an intervention of last resort.
  - Use caution when administering medications PRN for agitation or anxiety.
  - Determine the client's risk for injury, and ensure safety in the physical environment, such as a lowered bed.

Cognitive support

- Provide compensatory memory aids (clocks, calendars, photographs, memorabilia, seasonal decorations, familiar objects). Reorient as necessary.
- Keep a consistent daily routine.
- Maintain consistent caregivers.
- Cover or remove mirrors to decrease fear and agitation.
- Encourage physical activity during the day.
- Provide adequate lighting in the bathroom at night.

17.1 Delirium and neurocognitive disorder

	Delirium	Neurocognitive disorder
ONSET		
	Rapid over a short period of time (hours or days)	Gradual deterioration of function over months or years
MANIFESTATIONS		
	Impairments in memory, judgment, ability to focus, and ability to calculate, which can fluctuate throughout the day. Disorientation and confusion often worsen at night and early morning.	Impairments in memory, judgment, speech (aphasia), ability to recognize familiar objects (agnosia), executive functioning (managing daily tasks), and movement (apraxia); impairments do not change throughout the day.
	Level of consciousness is usually altered and can rapidly fluctuate.	Level of consciousness is usually unchanged.
	There are four types of delirium.	Restlessness and agitation are common; sundowning can occur.
	• Hyperactive with agitation and restlessness	Personality change is gradual.
	• Hypoactive with apathy and quietness	Vital signs are stable unless other illness is present.
	• Mixed, having a combination of hyper and hypo manifestations	
	• Unclassified for those whose manifestations do not classify into the other categories	
	Restlessness, anxiety, motor agitation, and fluctuating moods are common. Personality change is rapid.	
	Some perceptual disturbances can be present, such as hallucinations and illusions.	
	Change in reality can cause fear, panic, and anger.	
	Can cause vital signs to become unstable, requiring intervention	
	Should be considered a medical emergency	
CAUSE		
	Often associated with hospitalization of older adult clients	Cognitive deficits are not related to another mental health disorder.
	Medical conditions (infection) malnutrition, depression, electrolyte imbalance or substance use	Advanced age is the primary risk factor. Other causes include genetics, sedentary lifestyle, metabolic syndrome, and diabetes mellitus.
	Surgery, often secondary to withdrawal from illegal substances or alcohol, or impaired respiratory function	Subtypes of neurocognitive disorder can be related to:
		• Alzheimer's disease
		• Traumatic brain injury
		• Parkinson's disease
		• Other disorders affecting the neurologic system
OUTCOME		
	Reversible if diagnosis and treatment of underlying cause are prompt	Irreversible and progressive

Physical needs

- Monitor neurologic status.
- Identify disturbances in physiologic status, which can contribute to the cause of delirium.
- Check skin integrity, which can be compromised due to poor nutrition, bed rest, or incontinence.
- Monitor vital signs. Tachycardia, elevated blood pressure, sweating, and dilated pupils can be associated with delirium.
- Implement measures to promote sleep.
- Monitor the client's level of comfort and check for nonverbal indications of discomfort.
- Provide eyeglasses and assistive hearing devices as needed.
- Ensure adequate food and fluid intake. Underlying causes of delirium can result in electrolyte imbalance.

Communication

- Communicate in a calm, reassuring tone.
- Speak in positively worded phrases. Do not argue or question hallucinations or delusions.
- Reinforce reality.
- Reinforce orientation to time, place, and person.
- Introduce self to client with each new contact.
- Establish eye contact and use short, simple sentences when speaking to the client. Focus on one item of information at a time.
- Encourage reminiscence about happy times. Talk about familiar things.
- Break instructions and activities into short time frames.
- Limit the number of choices when dressing or eating.
- Minimize the need for decision-making and abstract thinking to avoid frustration.
- Avoid confrontation.
- Approach slowly and from the front. Address the client by name.
- Encourage family visitation as appropriate.

MEDICATIONS

Use caution when administering medications PRN for agitation or anxiety. Qs

Delirium

Medications can be the underlying cause of delirium. Recognize medication reactions before delirium occurs.
- Pharmacological management focuses on the treatment of the underlying disorder.
- Antipsychotic or antianxiety medications can be prescribed.

Neurocognitive disorders

Cholinesterase inhibitor medications (donepezil, rivastigmine, and galantamine) increase acetylcholine at cholinergic synapses by inhibiting its breakdown by acetylcholinesterase, which increases the availability of acetylcholine at neurotransmitter receptor sites in the CNS.

- In some clients, these medications improve the ability to perform self-care and slow cognitive deterioration of Alzheimer's disease in the mild to moderate stages.
- ADVERSE EFFECTS
  - GI effects: Nausea, vomiting, and diarrhea
    - Monitor for gastrointestinal adverse effects and for fluid volume deficits.
    - Promote adequate fluid intake.
    - The provider can titrate the dosage to reduce gastrointestinal effects.
  - Bradycardia, syncope
    - Instruct the family to monitor pulse rate for the client who lives at home.
    - The client should be screened for underlying heart disease.
- CONTRAINDICATIONS/PRECAUTIONS: Cholinesterase inhibitors should be used with caution in clients who have pre-existing asthma or other obstructive pulmonary disorders. Bronchoconstriction can be caused by an increase of acetylcholine.
- INTERACTIONS
  - **Concurrent use of NSAIDs (aspirin) can cause gastrointestinal bleeding.**
    - NURSING ACTIONS
      - Monitor the use of over-the-counter NSAIDs.
      - Monitor for indications of gastrointestinal bleeding.
  - **Antihistamines, tricyclic antidepressants, and conventional antipsychotics (medications that block cholinergic receptors) can reduce the therapeutic effects of donepezil.**
    - NURSING ACTIONS: Use of cholinergic receptor blocking medications for clients taking any cholinesterase inhibitor is not recommended.
- NURSING ADMINISTRATION
  - Dosage should start low and gradually be increased until adverse effects are no longer tolerable or medication is no longer beneficial.
  - Monitor for adverse effects, and educate the client and family about these effects. Taper medication when discontinuing to prevent abrupt progression of clinical manifestations. QEBP
  - Monitor the client for the ability to swallow tablets. Most medications are available in tablets and oral solutions. Donepezil is available in an orally disintegrating tablet.
  - Administer at bedtime with or without food.
  - Donepezil has a long half-life and is administered once daily at bedtime. The other cholinesterase inhibitors are usually administered twice daily.
  - Rivastigmine is available in oral form and as a patch that is applied once daily. Encourage clients to always take rivastigmine with food to reduce GI upset.

Medications (memantine) block the entry of calcium into nerve cells, thus slowing down brain-cell death.

- Memantine is approved for moderate to severe stages of AD.
- NURSING ACTIONS
  - Memantine can be used concurrently with a cholinesterase inhibitor.
  - Administer the medication with or without food.
  - Monitor for common adverse effects, including dizziness, headache, confusion, and constipation.

Other medications that may be prescribed include selective serotonin reuptake inhibitors for depression and antianxiety agents as needed for agitation. Antipsychotics are reserved for clients who experience hallucinations or delusions but are used as a last resort because these medications carry many adverse effects.

ALTERNATIVE/ COMPLEMENTARY THERAPIES

Some vitamins and herbal products are currently under investigation for the treatment of neurocognitive disorders. There is currently no evidence that these products are effective.

CLIENT EDUCATION

CARE AFTER DISCHARGE

- Educate family/caregivers about the client's illness, methods of care, and adaptation of the home environment.
- Ensure a safe environment in the home.

QUESTIONS TO ASK Qs

- Will the client wander out into the street if doors are left unlocked?
- Is the client able to remember their address and name?
- Does the client harm others when allowed to wander in a long-term care facility?

HOME SAFETY MEASURES Qs

- Remove scatter rugs.
- Install door locks that cannot be easily opened.
- Lock water heater thermostat and turn water temperature down to a safe level.
- Provide good lighting, especially on stairs.
- Install a handrail on stairs, and mark step edges with colored tape.
- Place mattresses on the floor.
- Remove clutter, keeping clear, wide pathways for walking through a room.
- Secure electrical cords to baseboards.
- Store cleaning supplies in locked cupboards.
- Install handrails in bathrooms.
- Allow for safe pacing and wandering.

SUPPORT FOR CAREGIVERS

- Encourage the client and family to seek legal counsel regarding advanced directives, guardianship, or durable power of attorney for health care.
- Determine teaching needs for the client and family members as the client's cognitive ability progressively declines.
- Review resources available to the family as the client's health declines. Include long-term care options. A variety of home care and community resources can be available in many areas of the country. These resources can allow the client to remain at home, rather than in a care facility. Qtc
- Provide support for caregivers. Encourage caregivers to ask for help from friends and other family members for respite care and to take advantage of local support groups.
- Encourage caregivers to take care of themselves and to take one day at a time.

Active Learning Scenario

A nurse is contributing to the plan of care to promote a safe and therapeutic environment for a client who has severe cognitive decline due to Alzheimer's disease. Use the ATI Active Learning Template: System Disorder to complete this item.

ALTERATIONS IN HEALTH (DIAGNOSIS)

NURSING CARE: Identify five nursing actions.

Active Learning Scenario Key

Using the ATI Active Learning Template: System Disorder

ALTERATIONS IN HEALTH (DIAGNOSIS): Alzheimer's disease is a subtype of neurocognitive disorder that is neurodegenerative, resulting in the gradual impairment of cognitive function. A client who has severe cognitive decline has memory difficulties, loss of awareness to recent events and surroundings, inability to recall personal history, personality changes, wandering behavior, the need for assistance with ADLs, disruption of sleep/wake cycle, and violent tendencies.

NURSING CARE
- Assign a room close to the nurses' station.
- Provide a room with a low level of visual and auditory stimuli.
- Provide for a well-lit environment, minimizing contrasts and shadows.
- Have the client sit in a room with windows to help with time orientation.
- Have the client wear an identification bracelet. Use monitors and bed alarm devices as needed.
- Monitor the client's level of comfort.
- Provide compensatory memory aids (clocks, calendars, photographs, memorabilia, seasonal decorations, and familiar objects). Reorient as necessary.
- Provide eyeglasses and assistive hearing devices as needed.
- Keep a consistent daily routine.
- Maintain consistent caregivers.
- Ensure adequate food and fluid intake.
- Allow for safe pacing and wandering.
- Cover or remove mirrors to decrease fear and agitation.

Ⓝ *NCLEX® Connection: Psychosocial Integrity, Therapeutic Environment*

1. A nurse is performing an admission assessment for a client who has delirium related to an acute urinary tract infection. Which of the following findings should the nurse expect? (Select all that apply.)

   A. History of gradual memory loss

   B. Family report of personality changes

   C. Hallucinations

   D. Unaltered level of consciousness

   E. Restlessness

2. A nurse is caring for a client who has early-stage Alzheimer's disease and a prescription for donepezil. The nurse should include which of the following statements when reinforcing teaching the client about the medication?

   A. "You should avoid taking over-the-counter acetaminophen while on donepezil."

   B. "You should take this medication before going to bed at the end of the day."

   C. "You will be screened for underlying kidney disease prior to starting donepezil."

   D. "You should stop taking donepezil if you experience nausea or diarrhea."

3. A nurse in a long-term care facility is caring for a client who has major neurocognitive disorder and attempts to wander out of the building. The client states, "I have to get home." Which of the following statements should the nurse make?

   A. "You have forgotten that this is your home."

   B. "You cannot go outside without a staff member."

   C. "Why would you want to leave? Aren't you happy with your care?"

   D. "I am your nurse. Let's walk together to your room."

4. A home health nurse is making a visit to a client who has Alzheimer's disease to collect data regarding the home for safety. Which of the following suggestions should the nurse make to decrease the client's risk for injury? (Select all that apply.)

   A. Install extra locks at the top of exit doors.

   B. Place rugs over electrical cords.

   C. Put cleaning supplies on the top of a shelf.

   D. Place the client's mattress on the floor.

   E. Install light fixtures above stairs.

5. A nurse is making a home visit to a client who is in the late stage of Alzheimer's disease. The client's partner, who is the primary caregiver, wishes to discuss concerns about the client's nutrition and the stress of providing care. Which of the following actions should the nurse take?

   A. Verify that a current power of attorney document is on file.

   B. Instruct the client's partner to offer finger foods to increase oral intake.

   C. Provide information on resources for respite care.

   D. Schedule the client for placement of an enteral feeding tube.

1. B, C, E. **CORRECT:** When recognizing cues, the nurse should identify the client who has delirium can experience rapid personality changes, perceptual disturbances (hallucinations and illusions), and restlessness and agitation. The client who has delirium can experience memory loss with sudden rather than gradual onset. The client who has delirium is expected to have an altered level of consciousness that can rapidly fluctuate. The client who has delirium commonly exhibits restlessness and agitation.

   Ⓝ *NCLEX® Connection: Psychosocial Integrity, Mental Health Concepts*

2. B. **CORRECT:** When taking action, the nurse should tell the client who has a prescription for donepezil to take it at the end of the day just before going to bed, with or without food. The nurse should tell the client to avoid NSAIDs, rather than acetaminophen, due to risk for gastrointestinal bleeding. Clients should be screened for underlying heart and pulmonary disease, rather than kidney disease, prior to treatment. Also, the nurse should instruct the client that gastrointestinal adverse effects are common with donepezil and can result in a dosage reduction. However, the client should not abruptly stop the medication without consulting a provider.

   Ⓝ *NCLEX® Connection: Pharmacological Therapies, Adverse Effects/Contraindications/Side Effects/Interactions*

3. D. **CORRECT:** When the nurse recognizes the client is attempting to wander out of the building, the nurse should introduce themselves with each new interaction and to promote reality in a calm, reassuring manner. Also, the nurse should avoid statements that can be interpreted as argumentative or demeaning. Using a "why" question can promote a defensive reaction and does not reinforce reality.

   Ⓝ *NCLEX® Connection: Psychosocial Integrity, Mental Health Concepts*

4. A, D, E. **CORRECT:** When taking action, the nurse should suggest the following to decrease the client's risk for injury in the home: placing door locks up high where they are difficult to reach to prevent exiting the home and wandering outside; placing the client's mattress on the floor to reduce the risk for falls out of the bed; and instructing the family to ensure there is adequate lighting around the stairs to reduce the risk for falls. Also, rugs create a fall risk hazard and should be removed. Electrical cords should be secured to baseboards rather than covered. Cleaning supplies should be placed in locked cupboards. Marking the supplies with colored tape does not prevent the client's access to hazardous materials.

   Ⓝ *NCLEX® Connection: Safety and Infection Control, Accident/ Error/Injury Prevention*

5. C. **CORRECT:** When discussing concerns about the client's nutrition and the stress of providing care, it is important to provide information on resources for respite care to allow the partner a break from caregiving responsibilities. A power of attorney document does not address the client's care or the concerns of the caregiver. Clients in late-stage Alzheimer's disease are at risk for choking and are unable to eat without assistance. Offering finger foods is not an appropriate action as there is no indication that the client is having difficulties using eating utensils. Placement of an enteral feeding tube is appropriate only with a prescription from the provider following a discussion that includes the provider, nurse, client's partner, and possibly social services and additional family members.

   Ⓝ *NCLEX® Connection: Management of Care, Referrals*

UNIT 3   PSYCHOBIOLOGIC DISORDERS

CHAPTER 18 *Substance Use and Addictive Disorders*

Substance use disorders are related to alcohol, caffeine, cannabis, hallucinogens, inhalants, opioids, sedatives/hypnotics/anxiolytics, stimulants, tobacco, and other (or unknown) substances.

A substance use disorder involves repeated use of chemical substances, leading to clinically significant impairment during a 12-month period. Non-substance-related disorders (behavioral/process addictions) include gambling, sexual activity, shopping, social media, and internet gaming.

Substance use and addictive disorders are characterized by loss of control due to the substance use or behavior, participation that continues despite continuing associated problems, and a tendency to relapse back into the substance use or behavior.

The defense mechanism of denial is commonly used by clients who have problems with a substance use or addictive disorder. For example, a person who has long-term tobacco use might say, "I can quit whenever I want to, but smoking really doesn't cause me any problems." Frequently, denial prevents a client from obtaining help with substance use or an addictive behavior.

DATA COLLECTION

RISK FACTORS

- Genetics: predisposition to developing a substance use disorder due to family history
- Adolescent population related to developing decision-making, judgment, and self-control skills
- Chronic stress: socioeconomic factors
- History of trauma: abuse, combat experience
- Lowered self-esteem

- Lowered tolerance for pain and frustration
- Few meaningful personal relationships
- Few life successes
- Risk-taking tendencies

PROTECTIVE FACTORS

- Positive family support, social relationships, and self-esteem
- Caregiver involvement in child and adolescent activities
- Availability of community resources and programs
- Employment

SOCIOCULTURAL THEORIES
- Some cultures (Alaska natives and Native American groups) have a high percentage of members who have alcohol use disorder. QEBP
  ○ Other cultures (Asian groups) have a low rate of alcohol use disorder.
  ○ Metabolism of alcohol and cultural views of alcohol use provide possible explanations for the incidence of alcohol use within a cultural group.
- Peer pressure and other sociological factors can increase the likelihood of substance use.
- Older adult clients can have a history of alcohol use or can develop a pattern of alcohol/substance use later in life due to life stressors (losing a partner or a friend, retirement, or social isolation). Ⓖ

EXPECTED FINDINGS

The nurse should use open-ended questions to obtain the following information for the nursing history. QPCC
- Type of substance or addictive behavior
- Pattern and frequency of substance use
- Amount of substance used
- Age at onset of substance use
- Changes in occupational or school performance
- Changes in use patterns
- Periods of abstinence in history
- Previous withdrawal manifestations
- Date of last substance use or addictive behavior

REVIEW OF SYSTEMS
- Blackout or loss of consciousness
- Changes in bowel movements
- Weight loss or weight gain
- Experience of stressful situations
- Sleep problems
- Chronic pain
- Concern over substance use
- Cutting down on consumption or behavior

POPULATION-SPECIFIC CONSIDERATIONS

- The rate of substance use is highest in clients who are 18 to 25 years of age.
- The younger the person is at the time of initial substance use, the higher the incidence of developing a substance use disorder.
- Cocaine use is decreased among adolescents. However, about half of adolescent population report access to marijuana.

- Substance use while pregnant creates risks for clients' infants, including an increased likelihood of prematurity, low birth weight, and neonatal abstinence syndrome.
- Health care providers are vulnerable to drug diversion.
  - Related to workplace stress and access to drugs
  - Concerning behaviors include volunteering for overtime, coming to work on days not working, deteriorating appearance and job performance, having mood swings, forgetting, and lying.
- Older adults who use substances are especially prone to falls and other injuries, memory loss, somatic reports (headaches), and changes in sleep patterns. Ⓖ
  - Indications of alcohol use in older adults can include a decrease in ability for self-care (functional status), urinary incontinence, and manifestations of dementia.
  - Older adults can show effects of alcohol use at lower doses than younger adults.
  - Polypharmacy (the use of multiple medications), the potential interaction between substances and medications, and age-related physiological changes raise the likelihood of adverse effects (confusion and falls) in older adult clients. QⱫ

STANDARDIZED SCREENING TOOLS

- Michigan Alcohol Screening Test (MAST) Qᴱᴮᴾ
- Drug Abuse Screening Test (DAST) or DAST-A: Adolescent version
- CAGE Questionnaire: Asks questions of clients to determine how they perceive their current alcohol use
- Alcohol Use Disorders Identification Test (AUDIT)
- Clinical Institute Withdrawal Assessment of Alcohol Scale, Revised (CIWA-Ar)
- Clinical Opiate Withdrawal Scale
- Screening, Brief Intervention, and Referral to Treatment (SBIRT)
  - Included in routine wellness screenings
  - Reduces risk drinking and related harms
  - Promotes safer drinking
  - Increases help-seeking among individuals who need it

COMMONLY USED SUBSTANCES

- Designer or club drugs (ecstasy) can combine substances from different categories, producing varying effects of intoxication or withdrawal.
- Improper use of prescription medications, specifically opioids, CNS depressants, and CNS stimulants, can result in substance use disorder and drug-seeking behavior.

OPIOID AGONISTS

Opioid agonists attach to CNS receptors, altering perception of and response to pain. This response can lead to generalized CNS depression. Prescribed opioid agonists are listed as Schedule II under the Controlled Substances Act.

Opioids

Heroin, morphine, and hydromorphone can be injected, smoked, inhaled, and swallowed. Misuse of prescription opioids for non-medical use has increased in the past few years.

INTENDED EFFECTS: A rush of euphoria, relief from pain

EFFECTS OF INTOXICATION
- Slurred speech, impaired memory, pupillary changes
- Decreased respirations and level of consciousness, which can cause death
- Maladaptive behavioral or psychological changes, including impaired judgment or social functioning
- An antidote, naloxone, available for IV use to relieve effects of toxicity

WITHDRAWAL MANIFESTATIONS
- Abstinence syndrome begins with sweating and rhinorrhea progressing to piloerection (gooseflesh), tremors, and irritability, followed by severe weakness, diarrhea, fever, insomnia, pupil dilation, nausea and vomiting, pain in the muscles and bones, and muscle spasms.
- Withdrawal is very unpleasant but not life-threatening.

CENTRAL NERVOUS SYSTEM DEPRESSANTS

CNS depressants can produce physiological and psychological dependence and can have cross-tolerance, cross-dependency, and an additive effect when taken concurrently.

Alcohol (ethanol)

- A laboratory blood alcohol concentration (BAC) of 0.08% (80 mg/dL) is considered legally intoxicated for adults operating automobiles in most U.S. states. Death could occur from acute toxicity in levels greater than about 0.4% (400 mg/dL).
- BAC depends on many factors, including body weight, gender, concentration of alcohol in drinks, number of drinks, gastric absorption rate, and the individual's tolerance level.
- Fetal alcohol syndrome symptoms include microcephaly, craniofacial malformations, and limb and heart defects, along with other developmental problems.

INTENDED EFFECTS: Relaxation, decreased social anxiety, stress reduction

EFFECTS OF INTOXICATION
- **Effects of excess:** Slurred speech, nystagmus, memory impairment, altered judgment, decreased motor skills, decreased level of consciousness (which can include stupor or coma), respiratory arrest, peripheral collapse, and death (with large doses)
- **Chronic use:** Direct cardiovascular damage, liver damage (ranging from fatty liver to cirrhosis), erosive gastritis and gastrointestinal bleeding, acute pancreatitis, sexual dysfunction

WITHDRAWAL MANIFESTATIONS

- Manifestations include abdominal cramping; vomiting; tremors; restlessness and inability to sleep; increased heart rate; transient hallucinations or illusions; anxiety; increased blood pressure, respiratory rate, and temperature; and tonic-clonic seizures.
- Alcohol withdrawal delirium can occur 2 to 3 days after cessation of alcohol. This is considered a medical emergency. Manifestations include severe disorientation, psychotic manifestations (hallucinations), severe hypertension, cardiac dysrhythmias, and delirium. Alcohol withdrawal delirium can progress to death.

Sedatives/hypnotics/anxiolytics

Benzodiazepines like diazepam, **barbiturates** like pentobarbital, or **club drugs** like flunitrazepam ("date rape drug") can be taken orally or injected.

INTENDED EFFECTS: Decreased anxiety, sedation

EFFECTS OF INTOXICATION

- Increased drowsiness and sedation, agitation, slurred speech, uncoordinated motor activity, nystagmus, disorientation, nausea, vomiting
- Respiratory depression and decreased level of consciousness, which can be fatal
- An antidote, flumazenil, available for IV use for benzodiazepine toxicity
- No antidote to reverse barbiturate toxicity

WITHDRAWAL MANIFESTATIONS: Anxiety, insomnia, diaphoresis, hypertension, possible psychotic reactions, hand tremors, nausea, vomiting, hallucinations or illusions, psychomotor agitation, and possible seizure activity

Cannabis

Marijuana or hashish (which is more potent) can be smoked or orally ingested.

INTENDED EFFECTS: Euphoria, sedation, hallucinations, decrease of nausea and vomiting secondary to chemotherapy, management of chronic pain

EFFECTS OF INTOXICATION

- Chronic use: increased risk for lung cancer and other respiratory effects; cannabis use disorder results in problems with performance of daily activities
- In high doses: occurrence of paranoia (delusions and hallucinations)
- Increased appetite, dry mouth, tachycardia
- Cannabis use can impair motor skills for 8 to 12 hr, impacting driving and use of machinery
- Synthetic cannabinoids, including K2 and Spice, have been associated with toxic doses. The chemicals are related to Marijuana but more potent.

WITHDRAWAL MANIFESTATIONS: Irritability, aggression, anxiety, insomnia, lack of appetite, restlessness, depressed mood, abdominal pain, tremors, diaphoresis, fever, headache

CENTRAL NERVOUS SYSTEM STIMULANTS

The CNS stimulation seen in some CNS stimulants is dependent on the area of the brain and spinal cord affected.

Cocaine

Can be injected, smoked, or inhaled (snorted)

INTENDED EFFECTS: Rush of euphoria (extreme well-being) and pleasure, increased energy

EFFECTS OF INTOXICATION

- **Mild toxicity:** dizziness, irritability, tremor, blurred vision
- **Severe effects:** hallucinations, seizures, extreme fever, tachycardia, hypertension, chest pain, possible cardiovascular collapse and death
- Nasal damage from inhaled cocaine

WITHDRAWAL MANIFESTATIONS

- Depression, fatigue, craving, excess sleeping or insomnia, dramatic unpleasant dreams, psychomotor retardation, agitation
- Not life-threatening, but possible occurrence of suicidal ideation

Amphetamines/methamphetamines

Can be taken orally, injected intravenously, snorted, or smoked

INTENDED EFFECTS: Increased energy, euphoria similar to cocaine

EFFECTS OF INTOXICATION

- Increased heart rate, blood pressure, body temperature, cardiac dysrhythmia, stroke, kidney failure, irritability, anxiety, panic, paranoia, psychosis
- Weight loss
- Heavy use can cause severe dental problems
- Prolonged deficits in cognition and memory
- Dilated pupils

WITHDRAWAL MANIFESTATIONS

- Craving, depression, fatigue, sleeping
- Not life-threatening

Inhalants

Amyl nitrate, nitrous oxide, and solvents are sniffed, huffed, or bagged, often by children or adolescents.

INTENDED EFFECTS: Euphoria

EFFECTS OF INTOXICATION: Depend on the substance, but generally can cause behavioral or psychological changes, dizziness, nystagmus, uncoordinated movements or gait, slurred speech, drowsiness, hyporeflexia, muscle weakness, diplopia, stupor or coma, respiratory depression, and possible death

WITHDRAWAL MANIFESTATIONS: None

Hallucinogens

Lysergic acid diethylamide (LSD), mescaline (peyote), and phencyclidine piperidine (PCP) are usually ingested orally, but can be injected or smoked.

INTENDED EFFECTS: Heightened sense of self and altered perceptions (colors being more vivid while under the influence)

EFFECTS OF INTOXICATION: Anxiety, depression, paranoia, impaired judgment, impaired social functioning, pupil dilation, tachycardia, diaphoresis, palpitations, blurred vision, tremors, incoordination, and panic attacks

WITHDRAWAL MANIFESTATIONS: **Hallucinogen persisting perception disorder:** Visual disturbances or flashback hallucinations can occur intermittently for years.

Caffeine

Includes cola drinks, coffee, tea, chocolate, energy drinks

INTENDED EFFECTS: Increased level of alertness and decreased fatigue

EFFECTS OF INTOXICATION: Intoxication commonly occurs with ingestion of greater than 250 mg. (One 2 oz high-energy drink can contain 215 to 240 mg caffeine.) Tachycardia and arrhythmias, flushed face, muscle twitching, restlessness, diuresis, GI disturbances, anxiety, insomnia

WITHDRAWAL MANIFESTATIONS
- Can occur within 24 hr of last consumption
- Headache, nausea, vomiting, muscle pain, irritability, inability to focus, drowsiness

OTHER

Nicotine affects nicotinic receptors in the brain, the carotid body, aortic arch, and CNS. Activation of these receptors can simulate the action that occurs with cocaine and other addictive substances.

Tobacco (nicotine)

- Cigarettes and cigars are inhaled.
- Smokeless tobacco is snuffed or chewed.

INTENDED EFFECTS: Relaxation, decreased anxiety

EFFECTS OF INTOXICATION
- Highly toxic, but acute toxicity seen only in children or when exposure is to nicotine in pesticides
- Also contains other harmful chemicals that are highly toxic and have long-term effects
- **Long-term effects**
  - Cardiovascular disease (hypertension, stroke), respiratory disease (emphysema, lung cancer)
  - With smokeless tobacco (snuff or "chew"): irritation to oral mucous membranes and cancer

WITHDRAWAL MANIFESTATIONS: Abstinence syndrome evidenced by irritability, craving, nervousness, restlessness, anxiety, insomnia, increased appetite, difficulty concentrating, anger, and depressed mood

PATIENT-CENTERED CARE

NURSING CARE

- Personal views, culture, and history can affect the nurse's feelings regarding substance use and addictive disorders. Nurse must self-assess their own feelings because those feelings can be transferred to clients through body language and the terminology nurses can use in data collection of clients. An objective, nonjudgmental nurse approach is imperative.
- Safety is the primary focus of nursing care during acute intoxication or withdrawal. Qs
  - Maintain a safe environment to prevent falls; implement seizure precautions as necessary.
  - Provide close observation for withdrawal manifestations, possibly one-on-one supervision. Physical restraint should be a last resort.
  - Orient the client to time, place, and person.
  - Maintain adequate nutrition and fluid balance.
  - Create a low-stimulation environment.
  - Administer medications as prescribed to treat the effects of intoxication or to prevent or manage withdrawal. This can include substitution therapy.
  - Monitor for covert substance use during the detoxification period.
- Provide emotional support and reassurance to the client and family. Educate the client and family about codependent behaviors.
- Reinforce teaching with the client and family about addiction and the initial treatment goal of abstinence.
- Reinforce teaching with the client and family regarding removing any prescription medications in the home that are not being used. Encourage the client not to share medication with someone for whom that medication is not prescribed.
- Begin to develop motivation and commitment for abstinence and recovery (abstinence plus developing a program of personal growth and self-discovery).
- Encourage self-responsibility.
- Help the client develop an emergency plan: a list of things the client would need to do and people they would need to contact.
- Encourage attendance at self-help groups.

INTERPROFESSIONAL CARE

Dual diagnosis, or comorbidity, means that an individual has both a mental health disorder (depression) and a substance use or addictive disorder. Both disorders need to be treated simultaneously and require a team approach.

Individual psychotherapies

- Cognitive behavioral therapies (relaxation techniques or cognitive reframing) can be used to decrease anxiety and change behavior.
- Acceptance and commitment therapy (ACT) promotes acceptance of the client's experiences and promotes client commitment to positive behavior changes.
- Relapse prevention therapy assists clients in identifying the potential for relapse and promotes behavioral self-control.

GROUP THERAPY: Groups of clients who have similar diagnoses can meet in an outpatient setting or within mental health residential facilities. Q_{TC}

Family therapy

- This therapy identifies codependency, which is a common behavior demonstrated by the significant other/family/friends of an individual with substance or process dependency and assists the family to change that behavior. The codependent person reacts in over-responsible ways that allow the dependent individual to continue the substance use or addiction disorder. For example, a partner can act as an enabler by calling the client's employer with an excuse of illness when the client is intoxicated.
- Families learn about use of specific substances.
- The client and family are educated regarding issues (family coping, problem-solving, indications of relapse, and availability of support groups). Q_{PCC}

CLIENT EDUCATION

- Instruct the client to recognize indications of relapse and factors that contribute to relapse.
- Reinforce cognitive-behavioral techniques to help maintain sobriety and create feelings of pleasure from activities other than using substances or from process addictions.
- Assist the client to develop communication skills to communicate with co-workers and family members while sober.
- Encourage the client and family to attend a 12-step program (Alcoholics Anonymous [AA], Narcotics Anonymous, Gambler's Anonymous), and family groups (Al-Anon, Ala-Teen). Q_{EBP}
  - These programs will teach clients the following.
    - Abstinence is necessary for recovery.
    - A higher power is needed to assist in recovery.
    - Clients are not responsible for their disease but are responsible for their recovery.
    - Other people cannot be blamed for the client's addictions, and they must acknowledge their feelings and problems.

18.1 Case study

Scenario introduction

A nurse in a local community mental health clinic is assisting with planning care and reviewing the medical record of a client who has been involuntarily committed to outpatient treatment services following a recent arrest for public intoxication. Following review of the client's medical record, the nurse and provider are discussing the client's status and treatment plan.

Scene 1

Provider: "Please provide me with a brief history regarding the client."

Nurse: "Sure. The client has an axis I diagnosis of major depressive disorder and an axis II diagnosis of substance use disorder. The client reports recently losing their job and recently separating from their partner. The client was in a medication assisted program for a history of substance use disorder following a car crash 10 years ago. The client has been referred to treatment because of relapse and use of opioids over the past month. Also, the client was arrested due to alcohol and opioid intoxication and court-ordered to treatment."

Scene 2

Provider: "What types of barriers is the client encountering that are making it difficult for them to adhere to the treatment program?"

Nurse: "The client lost their job recently, resulting in financial stress and transportation issues, and now they are uninsured."

Scenario conclusion

After collaborating with the provider, the nurse continues to assist with developing a plan of care for the client to identify actions to support the client.

Case study exercises

1. Identify the client's socioeconomic factors that could impact their social determinants of health (SDOH).

2. What questions should the nurse ask the client to identify any social determinants of health concerns?

3. Name some community partnerships related to SDOH the mental health nurses can explore when assisting the client.

Medications for substance use disorders

Abstinence syndrome occurs when a client abruptly withdraws from a substance on which they are physically dependent.

Clients who have a substance use disorder can experience tolerance and withdrawal. Tolerance occurs when a client requires increased amounts of the substance to achieve the desired effect. Withdrawal occurs when the concentration of the substance in the client's bloodstream declines and the client experiences physiological adverse effects. Withdrawing from a substance that has the potential to cause abstinence syndrome can cause the client to experience distressing manifestations that are potentially life-threatening.

WITHDRAWAL MANIFESTATIONS

Alcohol

- Manifestations usually start within 4 to 12 hr of the last intake of alcohol and can continue 5 to 7 days.
- Common manifestations include nausea; vomiting; tremors; restlessness and inability to sleep; depressed mood or irritability; increased heart rate, blood pressure, respiratory rate, and temperature; diaphoresis; tonic-clonic seizures; and illusions.
- Alcohol withdrawal delirium can occur 2 to 3 days after cessation of alcohol. This is considered a medical emergency. Manifestations include severe disorientation, psychotic effects (hallucinations), severe hypertension, and cardiac dysrhythmias. This type of withdrawal can progress to death. Qs

Opioids

- Withdrawal manifestations occur within hours to several days after cessation of opioid use.
- Common findings include agitation, insomnia, flu-like manifestations, rhinorrhea, yawning, sweating, nausea or vomiting, pupillary dilation, and diarrhea.
- Withdrawal manifestations are not life-threatening, but suicidal ideation can occur.

Tobacco (nicotine)

Abstinence syndrome is evidenced by irritability, nervousness, restlessness, insomnia, and difficulty concentrating.

Other substances associated with substance use disorder include cannabis, hallucinogens, inhalants, sedatives/hypnotics, and stimulants.

Alcohol

WITHDRAWAL

Benzodiazepines

- Chlordiazepoxide
- Diazepam
- Lorazepam
- Oxazepam

INTENDED EFFECTS
- Maintenance of vital signs within expected reference ranges
- Decrease in the risk of seizures
- Decrease in the intensity of withdrawal manifestations
- Substitution therapy during alcohol withdrawal

NURSING ACTIONS
- Administer around-the-clock or PRN as prescribed.
- Obtain baseline vital signs.
- Monitor vital signs and neurologic status on an ongoing basis.
- Assist with initiating for seizure precautions.

Adjunct medications

- Carbamazepine
- Clonidine
- Propranolol
- Atenolol

INTENDED EFFECTS
- Reduction of manifestations of withdrawal and decrease in seizures: Carbamazepine
- Depression of autonomic response (decrease in blood pressure, heart rate): Clonidine, propranolol, atenolol
- Decrease in craving: Propranolol, atenolol

NURSING ACTIONS
- Implement seizure precautions. Qs
- Obtain baseline vital signs and continue to monitor.
- Check heart rate prior to administration of beta blockers, and withhold if less than 50/min.

ABSTINENCE MAINTENANCE (FOLLOWING WITHDRAWAL)

Disulfiram

INTENDED EFFECTS
- Disulfiram is a daily oral medication that is a type of aversion (behavioral) therapy.
- Disulfiram used concurrently with even small amounts of alcohol will cause acetaldehyde syndrome to occur. Effects include nausea, vomiting, weakness, sweating, palpitations, and hypotension. Acetaldehyde syndrome can progress to respiratory depression, cardiovascular suppression, seizures, and death. Qs

NURSING ACTIONS
- Monitor liver function tests to detect hepatotoxicity.
- First dose should not be administered until 12 hr after the last drink.

CLIENT EDUCATION

- Drinking any alcohol is potentially dangerous.
- Avoid use or contact with any products that contain alcohol (cough syrup, aftershave lotion, mouthwash, hand sanitizer).
- Wear a medical alert bracelet.
- Participate in a self-help program. ⓠpcc
- Medication effects (the potential for acetaldehyde syndrome with alcohol ingestion) persist for 2 weeks following discontinuation of disulfiram.

Naltrexone

INTENDED EFFECTS

- Naltrexone is a pure opioid antagonist that suppresses the craving and pleasurable effects of alcohol and prevents relapse in the recovery phase.
- Detoxification; maintenance
- Complete opioid antagonist to prevent narcotic effects

NURSING ACTIONS

- Collect data about the client's history to determine whether the client is also dependent on opioids. Concurrent use increases the risk for opioid toxicity.
- Suggest monthly IM injections of depot naltrexone for clients who have difficulty adhering to the medication regimen.

CLIENT EDUCATION

- Take naltrexone with meals to decrease gastrointestinal distress.
- Concurrent use of heroin can cause withdrawal manifestations and death. ⓠs

Acamprosate

INTENDED EFFECTS: Acamprosate is taken orally three times a day to reduce the unpleasant effects of abstinence (dysphoria, anxiety, restlessness).

CLIENT EDUCATION

- Diarrhea can result. Maintain adequate fluid intake to prevent dehydration.
- Avoid with kidney impairment.

Opioids

Methadone substitution

INTENDED EFFECTS

- Methadone substitution is an oral opioid agonist that replaces the opioid to which the client has a physical dependence.
- Methadone administration prevents abstinence syndrome from occurring and removes the need for the client to obtain illegal opioids.
- Methadone substitution is used for withdrawal and long-term maintenance.
- Dependence is transferred from the illegal opioid to methadone.

NURSING ACTIONS

- Encourage the client to participate in a 12-step program.
- Inform clients that the methadone dose must be slowly tapered to produce detoxification.
- Inform the client that the medication must be administered from an approved treatment center.

Clonidine

INTENDED EFFECTS

- Clonidine assists with opioid withdrawal effects related to autonomic hyperactivity (diarrhea, nausea, vomiting).
- Clonidine therapy does not reduce the craving for opioids.

NURSING ACTIONS

- Obtain baseline vital signs.
- Monitor for manifestations of opioid withdrawal (elevated vital signs, nausea, vomiting, diarrhea, yawning, runny nose, and goose bumps).

CLIENT EDUCATION

- Avoid activities that require mental alertness until drowsiness subsides.
- Chew sugarless gum, suck on hard candy, and sip small amounts of water to treat dry mouth.

Naltrexone

INTENDED EFFECTS

- Naltrexone is a full opioid antagonist.
- This medication is used to prevent relapse after opioid detoxification.
- If an opioid is used concurrently with naltrexone, the pleasurable effects will be blocked.

NURSING ACTIONS: Routes include oral daily doses or monthly intramuscular injections.

Buprenorphine

INTENDED EFFECTS

- Buprenorphine is an agonist-antagonist opioid used for both withdrawal and maintenance.
- This medication decreases feelings of craving and can be effective in maintaining compliance.
- FDA has approved a variety of schedule III buprenorphine products, some containing naloxone, and are available as sublingual tablets, buccal film, and a surgical skin implant.

NURSING ACTIONS

- Unlike methadone, a primary care provider can prescribe and dispense buprenorphine.
- Administer the medication sublingually.

Antidotes

- Naloxone: A specific opioid antagonist, can be given IM, SQ, IV or via inhalation, to reverse respiratory depression, coma, and other effects of opioid toxicity.
- Flumazenil: Competitive benzodiazepine receptor antagonist, can reverse sedative effects and toxicity. Administered IV

INTENDED EFFECTS
- Competes with and blocks opioid receptor to prevent action of narcotic
- Used in overdose situations

Nicotine

Bupropion

INTENDED EFFECTS: Bupropion decreases nicotine craving and manifestations of withdrawal.

CLIENT EDUCATION
- To treat dry mouth, chew sugarless gum, suck on ice chips or hard candy, and sip on small amounts of water.
- Avoid caffeine and other CNS stimulants to control insomnia.

Nicotine replacement therapy

Nicotine gum, nicotine patch, nicotine nasal spray, nicotine lozenges, nicotine inhaler

INTENDED EFFECTS
- Nicotine replacements are pharmaceutical product substitutes for the nicotine in cigarettes or chewing tobacco.
- The rate of tobacco use cessation is nearly doubled with the use of nicotine replacements. Q EBP
- Nicotine inhaler simulates smoking because the client puffs on the inhaler, which delivers nicotine.

NURSING ACTIONS
- Nasal spray provides pleasurable effects of smoking due to rapid rise of the nicotine level in the client's blood.
- One spray in each nostril delivers the amount of nicotine in one cigarette.
- Nicotine nasal spray is not recommended for clients who have disorders affecting the upper respiratory system (chronic sinus problems, allergies, or asthma).
- Contains menthol, which creates sensation in the back of the throat similar to smoking
- Avoid the use of nicotine inhalers in clients who have asthma.
- Gradually taper nicotine inhaler use over 2 to 3 months and then discontinue.

CLIENT EDUCATION
- **Nicotine gum**
  - Chew nicotine gum slowly and intermittently over 30 min.
  - Avoid eating or drinking 15 min prior to and while chewing nicotine gum.
  - Use of nicotine gum is not recommended for longer than 6 months.
- **Nicotine patch**
  - Apply a nicotine patch to an area of clean, dry skin each day.
  - Follow directions for dosage times. In general, nicotine patches are applied in the morning and removed 16 hr later at bedtime.
  - Nightmares or sleep disturbance have been reported when wearing patches during the night.
  - Avoid using any nicotine products while wearing the patch.
  - Remove the nicotine patch and notify the provider if a local skin reaction occurs.
  - Remove the nicotine patch prior to magnetic resonance imaging (MRI).
- **Nicotine spray**
  - One spray in each nostril delivers the amount of nicotine in one cigarette.
  - Follow product instructions for dosage of nasal spray frequency.
- **Nicotine lozenges**
  - Avoid oral intake 15 min prior to or during nicotine lozenge use.
  - Allow nicotine lozenges to slowly dissolve in the mouth (20 to 30 min).
  - Follow product directions for dosage strength and recommended titration.
  - Limit lozenge use to five in a 6-hr period or a maximum of 20/day.

Varenicline

INTENDED EFFECTS: Varenicline is a nicotinic receptor agonist that promotes the release of dopamine to simulate the pleasurable effects of nicotine.

- Reduces cravings for nicotine as well as the severity of withdrawal manifestations
- Reduces the incidence of relapse by blocking the desired effects of nicotine

NURSING ACTIONS
- Monitor blood pressure during treatment.
- Monitor clients who have diabetes mellitus for loss of glycemic control.
- Follow instructions for titration to minimize adverse effects.
- Due to potential adverse effects, varenicline is banned for use in clients who are commercial truck or bus drivers, air traffic controllers, or airplane pilots.
- Warn client of cardiovascular risks and the need to seek immediate attention for chest pain.

CLIENT EDUCATION
- Instruct the client to take medication after a meal.
- Notify the provider if persistent nausea, vomiting, insomnia, new-onset depression, or suicidal thoughts occur.
- Monitor for neuropsychiatric effects (unpredictable behavior, mood changes, and thoughts of suicide).
- Can cause mild to moderate nausea

Electronic cigarettes (e-cigarettes)

Use of electronic-cigarettes (e-cigarettes) should be discouraged due to their dose of nicotine being unpredictable, and data on safety and efficacy are lacking. Qs

NURSING EVALUATION OF MEDICATION EFFECTIVENESS

Depending on therapeutic intent, effectiveness can be evidenced by the following.
- Absence of injury
- Ongoing abstinence from the substance
- Regular attendance at a 12-step program
- Decreased cravings for substance
- Improved coping skills to replace use of substance

Active Learning Scenario

A nurse is caring for a client who has cocaine use disorder and is experiencing severe effects of intoxication. Use the ATI Active Learning Template: System Disorder to complete this item.

ALTERATIONS IN HEALTH (DIAGNOSIS)

EXPECTED FINDINGS: Identify three expected findings.

NURSING CARE: Describe two nursing interventions.

INTERPROFESSIONAL CARE: Describe two forms of nonpharmacological therapy.

CLIENT EDUCATION: Identify two client outcomes.

Application Exercises

1. A nurse is assisting with a staff education program on substance use in older adults. Which of the following information should the nurse include in the presentation?
   A. Older adults require higher doses of a substance to achieve a desired effect.
   B. Older adults commonly use rationalization to cope with a substance use disorder.
   C. Older adults are at an increased risk for substance use following retirement.
   D. Older adults develop substance use to mask manifestations of dementia.

2. A nurse is caring for a client who has alcohol use disorder and is experiencing withdrawal. Which of the following findings should the nurse expect? (Select all that apply.)
   A. Bradycardia
   B. Fine tremors of both hands
   C. Decreased blood pressure
   D. Vomiting
   E. Restlessness

3. A nurse is contributing to the plan of care for a client who is experiencing benzodiazepine withdrawal. Which of the following interventions should the nurse identify as the priority?
   A. Orient the client frequently to time, place, and person.
   B. Offer fluids and nourishing diet as tolerated.
   C. Implement seizure precautions.
   D. Encourage participation in group therapy sessions.

4. A nurse is caring for a client who has alcohol use disorder. The client is no longer experiencing withdrawal manifestations. Which of the following medications should the nurse anticipate administering to assist the client with maintaining abstinence from alcohol?
   A. Chlordiazepoxide
   B. Bupropion
   C. Disulfiram
   D. Carbamazepine

5. A nurse is reinforcing teaching with the family of a client who has a substance use disorder. Which of the following statements by a family member indicates an understanding of the instruction? (Select all that apply.)
   A. "We need to understand that our sibling is responsible for their disorder."
   B. "Eliminating codependent behavior will promote recovery."
   C. "Our sibling should participate in an Al-Anon group to assist with recovery."
   D. "The primary goal of treatment is abstinence from substance use."
   E. "Our sibling needs to discuss personal feelings about substance use to help with recovery."

6. A nurse is assisting in the discharge planning for a client following alcohol detoxification. The nurse should expect prescriptions for which of the following medications to promote long-term abstinence from alcohol? (Select all that apply.)
   A. Lorazepam
   B. Diazepam
   C. Disulfiram
   D. Naltrexone
   E. Acamprosate

Application Exercises Key

1. C. **CORRECT:** Retirement and other life change stressors increase the risk for substance use in older adults, especially if there is a prior history of substance use. Requiring higher doses of a substance to achieve a desired effect is a result of the length and severity of substance use rather than age. Denial, rather than rationalization, is a defense mechanism commonly used by substance users of all ages. Substance use in the older adult can result in manifestations of dementia.

   (N) *NCLEX® Connection: Psychosocial Integrity, Chemical and Other Dependencies/Substance Use Disorder*

2. B, D, E. **CORRECT:** Fine tremors of both hands are an expected finding of alcohol withdrawal. Vomiting is an expected finding of alcohol withdrawal. Restlessness is an expected finding of alcohol withdrawal. An expected finding of alcohol withdrawal is tachycardia rather than bradycardia. An expected finding of alcohol withdrawal is hypertension rather than hypotension.

   (N) *NCLEX® Connection: Psychosocial Integrity, Chemical and Other Dependencies/Substance Use Disorder*

3. C. **CORRECT:** The greatest risk to the client is injury. Implementing seizure precautions is the priority intervention. Reorienting the client is an appropriate intervention. However, it is not the priority. Providing hydration and nourishment is an appropriate intervention. However, it is not the priority. Encouraging participation in therapy is an appropriate intervention. However, it is not the priority.

   (N) *NCLEX® Connection: Safety and Infection Control, Accident/ Error/Injury Prevention*

4. C. **CORRECT:** The nurse should expect to administer disulfiram to help the client maintain abstinence from alcohol. Chlordiazepoxide is indicated for acute alcohol withdrawal rather than to maintain abstinence from alcohol. Bupropion is indicated for nicotine withdrawal rather than to maintain abstinence from alcohol. Carbamazepine is indicated for acute alcohol withdrawal rather than to maintain abstinence from alcohol.

   (N) *NCLEX® Connection: Pharmacological Therapies, Expected Actions/Outcomes*

5. B, D, E. **CORRECT:** Families should be aware of codependent behavior (enabling) that can promote substance use rather than recovery. Abstinence is the primary treatment goal for a client who has a substance use disorder. Clients must acknowledge their feelings about substance use as part of a substance use recovery program. Al-Anon is a recovery group for the family of a client, rather than the client who has a substance use disorder. Clients are not responsible for their disease but are responsible for their recovery.

   (N) *NCLEX® Connection: Psychosocial Integrity, Chemical and Other Dependencies/Substance Use Disorder*

6. A. Lorazepam is prescribed for short-term use during withdrawal.
   B. Diazepam is prescribed for short-term use during withdrawal.
   C. **CORRECT:** Disulfiram promotes abstinence through aversion therapy.
   D. **CORRECT:** Naltrexone promotes abstinence by suppressing the craving and pleasurable effects of alcohol.
   E. **CORRECT:** Acamprosate decreases the unpleasant effects resulting from abstinence.

   (N) *NCLEX® Connection: Psychosocial Integrity, Chemical and Other Dependencies/Substance Use Disorder*

Case Study Exercises Key

1. When analyzing cues, the nurse should recognize that the client is currently unemployed and uninsured, which could impact overall health. Also, the client has an impaired support system and recent arrest for alcohol and opioid intoxication.

2. Do you have any close relatives who used substances of any kind when you were growing up? Does using the substance cause you problems? Have you ever been arrested for substance use? Do you have any transportation concerns? Describe a typical day in your life.

3. When generating solutions, the nurse recognizes that possible community partnerships include asking for peer support groups within the community, referring the client to a medication assisted treatment program, and providing education about 12-step recovery programs and financial and legal assistance.

Active Learning Scenario Key

Using the ATI Active Learning Template: System Disorder

ALTERATIONS IN HEALTH (DIAGNOSIS): Cocaine use disorder involves the repeated use of cocaine, leading to clinically significant impairment over a 12-month period.

EXPECTED FINDINGS
- Objective: Seizures, extreme fever, tachycardia, hypertension
- Subjective: Hallucinations, chest pain

NURSING CARE
- Perform a nursing self-assessment.
- Maintain a safe environment.
- Implement seizure precautions.
- Orient the client to time, place, and person.
- Create a low-stimulation environment.
- Monitor the client's vital signs and neurologic status.

INTERPROFESSIONAL CARE
- Cognitive behavioral therapies decrease anxiety and promote a change in behavior.
- Acceptance and commitment therapy promotes acceptance of the client and promotes a commitment to change.
- Relapse prevention therapy assists clients in identifying relapse and promotes self-control.
- Group therapy allows clients who have similar diagnoses to work together toward recovery.
- Family therapy allows the client and family members to work together toward recovery.
- Narcotics Anonymous provides a 12-step program to promote recovery and abstinence from future substance use.

CLIENT EDUCATION: Client outcomes
- The client will verbalize coping strategies to use in times of stress.
- The client will remain substance-free.
- The client will remain free from injury.
- The client will attend a 12-step program regularly.

(N) *NCLEX® Connection: Psychosocial Integrity, Chemical and Other Dependencies/Substance Use Disorder*

CHAPTER 19

Eating disorders describe a complex set of behaviors related to eating and share many similarities to anxiety-related disorders. Clients with eating disorders describe feeling out of control in other areas of their lives and use food as a coping mechanism. They may also have distorted perceptions of what they look like, which affects how they feel about themselves.

The exact prevalence and incidence of eating disorders existing in a given population during a designated time are most likely underestimated because of the secretiveness of the condition, denial that the illness exists, or avoidance of seeking professional help. The mortality rate for eating disorders is high, and suicide is also a risk.

Treatment modalities focus on normalizing eating patterns and beginning to address the issues raised by the illness. Q EBP

Comorbidities include depression, personality disorders, substance use disorder, and anxiety. Various eating disorders are recognized and defined by the DSM-5-TR.

Anorexia nervosa

- Persistent energy intake restriction leading to significantly low body weight in context of age, sex, developmental path, and physical health
- Fear of gaining weight or becoming overweight
- Disturbance in self-perceived weight or shape

CHARACTERISTICS
- Clients are preoccupied with food and the rituals of eating, along with a voluntary refusal to eat.
- This condition occurs most often in female clients from adolescence to young adulthood.
- Onset can be associated with a stressful life event, such as college.
- Compared with clients who have restricting type, those who have binge-eating/purging type have higher rates of impulsivity and are more likely to abuse drugs and alcohol.

TYPES
- **Restricting type:** The individual drastically restricts food intake and does not binge or purge.
- **Binge-eating/purging type:** The individual engages in binge eating or purging behaviors.

Bulimia nervosa

- Clients recurrently eat large quantities of food over a short period of time (binge eating), which can be followed by inappropriate compensatory behaviors (self-induced vomiting [purging]), to rid the body of the excess calories.
- Binge eating and inappropriate compensatory behavior both occur on average of once per week for 3 months.
- Binge eating is in a discrete period of time (usually less than 2 hours), and an amount of food definitely larger than what most individuals would eat in a similar period of time. Clients have a sense of lack of control over eating.

CHARACTERISTICS
- Most clients who have bulimia nervosa maintain a weight within a normal range or slightly higher. BMI is 18.5 to 30.
- The average age of onset in female clients is late adolescence or early adulthood.
- Bulimia nervosa occurs most commonly in female clients.
- Between binges, clients typically restrict caloric intake and select low-calorie "diet" foods.

TYPES
- **Purging type:** The client uses self-induced vomiting, laxatives, diuretics, and/or enemas to lose or maintain weight.
- **Nonpurging type:** The client can compensate for binge eating through other means (excessive exercise and the misuse of laxatives, diuretics, and/or enemas).

Binge eating disorder

- Clients recurrently eat large quantities of food over a short period of time without the use of compensatory behaviors associated with bulimia nervosa.
- Clients experience distress following the binge-eating episode.
- An excessive food consumption must be accompanied by a sense of lack of control.
- At least once per week for 3 months
- Binge eating is the most common eating disorder and is highest in adult females.
- The weight gain associated with binge eating disorder increases the client's risk for other disorders, including type 2 diabetes mellitus, hypertension, and cancer.
- Severity of the disorder depends on the number of binge-eating episodes each week.

Additional eating disorder categories

- **Pica:** Eating nonfood items like dirt, soap, or paint chips as if they were food
- **Rumination disorder:** Regurgitating food after eating it (Behaviors may be referred to as "chewing and spitting.")
- **Avoidant/restrictive food intake disorder:** a lack of interest in eating certain types of food, which leads to poor growth and nutrition

PRODROMAL MANIFESTATIONS

- Increase or decrease in weight that is not related to a medical condition
- Abnormal eating habits, like severe dieting
- Ritualized mealtime behaviors, like counting calories
- Lying about food intake
- Preoccupation with weight and body image
- Compulsive and/or excessive exercising

DATA COLLECTION

RISK FACTORS

- Occupational choices that encourage thinness (fashion modeling)
- Individual history of being a "picky" eater in childhood
- Participation in athletics, especially at an elite level of competition or in a sport where lean body build is prized (bicycling) or where a specific weight is necessary (wrestling)
- A history of obesity

FAMILY GENETICS: more commonly seen in families who have a history of eating disorders

BIOLOGICAL: hypothalamic, neurotransmitter, hormonal, or biochemical imbalance, with disturbances of the serotonin neurotransmitter pathways seeming to be implicated

INTERPERSONAL RELATIONSHIPS: influenced by parental pressure and the need to succeed

PSYCHOLOGICAL INFLUENCES: rigidity, ritualism; separation and individuation conflicts; feelings of ineffectiveness, helplessness, and depression; distorted body image; internal or external locus of control or self-identity; and potential history of physical abuse

ENVIRONMENTAL FACTORS: media influence and pressure from society to have the "perfect body"

TEMPERAMENTAL: anxiety or obsessional traits in childhood

EXPECTED FINDINGS

Nursing history should include the following. ⓠPCC
- The client's perception of the issue
- Eating habits
- History of dieting
- Methods of weight control (restricting, purging, exercising)
- Value attached to a specific shape and weight
- Interpersonal and social functioning
- Difficulty with impulsivity, as well as compulsivity
- Family and interpersonal relationships (frequently troublesome and chaotic, reflecting a lack of nurturing)

MENTAL STATUS
- Cognitive distortions include the following.
  - **Overgeneralizations:** "Other people don't like me because I'm fat."
  - **"All-or-nothing" thinking:** "If I eat any dessert, I'll gain 50 pounds."
  - **Catastrophizing:** "My life is over if I gain weight."
  - **Personalization:** "When I walk through the hospital hallway, I know everyone is looking at me."
  - **Emotional reasoning:** "I know I look bad because I feel bloated."
- Client demonstrates high interest in preparing food but not eating.
- Client is terrified of gaining weight.
- Client perception is that they are severely overweight and sees this image reflected in the mirror.
- Client can exhibit low self-esteem, impulsivity, and difficulty with interpersonal relationships.
- Client can exhibit the need for an intense physical regimen.
- Client can experience guilt or shame due to binge eating behavior.
- Obsessive-compulsive features can be related and unrelated to food (collecting recipes, hoarding food, concerns about eating in public).

VITAL SIGNS
- Low blood pressure with possible orthostatic hypotension
- Decreased pulse and body temperature
- Hypertension can be present in clients who have binge-eating disorder.

WEIGHT: Clients who have anorexia nervosa have a body weight that is less than 85% of expected normal weight.
- Most clients who have bulimia nervosa maintain a weight within the normal range or slightly higher.
- Clients who have binge eating disorder are typically overweight or obese.

SKIN, HAIR, AND NAILS
- Clients who have anorexia nervosa can have fine, downy hair (lanugo) on the face and back; yellowed skin; pale, cool extremities; and poor skin turgor.
- Clients who engage in purging activities can have calluses or scars on the hand (Russell's sign).

HEAD, NECK, MOUTH, AND THROAT
- Clients who engage in purging activities can have enlargement of the parotid glands.
- Dental erosion and caries (if the client is purging)

CARDIOVASCULAR SYSTEM
- Irregular heart rate (dysrhythmias noted on cardiac monitor), heart failure, cardiomyopathy
- Peripheral edema
- Acrocyanosis

FLUID/ELECTROLYTE
- Acidosis or alkalosis
- Dehydration
- Electrolyte imbalances

MUSCULOSKELETAL SYSTEM
- Muscle weakness
- Decreased energy
- Loss of bone density

GASTROINTESTINAL SYSTEM
- Constipation (dehydration)
- Diarrhea (laxative use)
- Abdominal pain
- Self-induced vomiting
- Excessive use of diuretics or laxatives
- Esophageal tears, gastric rupture (bulimia)

REPRODUCTIVE STATUS
- Amenorrhea can be seen in clients who have anorexia nervosa.
- Menstrual irregularities

PSYCHOSOCIAL
- Client can exhibit low self-esteem, impulsivity, and difficulty with interpersonal relationships.
- Depressed mood
- Social withdrawal
- Irritability
- Insomnia

CRITERIA FOR ACUTE CARE TREATMENT

- Rapid weight loss or weight loss of greater than 30% of body weight over 6 months
- Unsuccessful weight gain in outpatient treatment, failure to adhere to treatment contract
- Vital signs demonstrating heart rate less than 40/min, systolic blood pressure less than 70 mm Hg, body temperature less than 36° C (96.8° F)
- ECG changes
- Electrolyte disturbances
- Psychiatric criteria: severe depression, suicidal behavior, family crisis, or psychosis Qs

LABORATORY AND DIAGNOSTIC TESTS

COMMON LABORATORY ABNORMALITIES ASSOCIATED WITH ANOREXIA AND BULIMIA
- Hypokalemia, especially for those who have bulimia nervosa Qs
  ○ There is a direct loss of potassium due to purging (vomiting) and starvation.
  ○ Dehydration stimulates increased aldosterone production, which leads to sodium and water retention and potassium excretion.

- Anemia and leukopenia with lymphocytosis; thrombocytopenia
- Possible impaired liver function, evidenced by increased enzyme levels
- Hypoalbuminemia
- Possible elevated cholesterol
- Elevated blood urea nitrogen (dehydration)
- Abnormal thyroid function tests
- Elevated carotene levels, which cause skin to appear yellow
- Decreased bone density (possible osteoporosis)
- Abnormal blood glucose level
- ECG changes (prolonged QT interval)
- Possible increase of blood bicarbonate (metabolic alkalosis) related to self-induced vomiting
- Possible decrease of blood bicarbonate (metabolic acidosis) related to laxative use

---

19.1 Case study

Scenario introduction

A nurse is discussing anorexia nervosa and expected findings associated with the disorder with a newly licensed nurse.

Scene 1

Ian: "It is important to understand the expected findings associated with anorexia nervosa. What do you know about this eating disorder?"

Carla (with hesitation and apprehension): "Uh, let me think about it. I often get the signs and symptoms of anorexia and bulimia mixed up."

Ian: "Carla, you may want to list them out on a piece of paper and see if that helps you have a better understanding of the manifestations of the disorders."

Scene 2

Carla: "Sounds like a good idea."

Scenario conclusion

Carla should have an understanding of anorexia nervosa and the expected findings associated with the disorder.

Case Study Exercises

1. Identify and sort the expected findings associated with anorexia nervosa or bulimia nervosa.

   A. Dental erosion

   B. Severe dieting

   C. Loss of bone density

   D. Fear of gaining weight

   E. Esophageal tears

   F. Amenorrhea

   G. Menstrual irregularities

2. The nurse should identify which of the following electrolyte imbalances are associated with anorexia nervosa? (Select all that apply.)

   A. Hypokalemia

   B. Hypermagnesemia

   C. Hyponatremia

   D. Hypochloremia

   E. Hypophosphatemia

Electrolyte imbalances can depend on the client's method of purging (laxatives, diuretics, vomiting).
- Hypokalemia
- Hyponatremia
- Hypochloremia
- Hypomagnesemia (occurs due to malnutrition)
- Hypophosphatemia (occurs due to malnutrition)
- Decreased estrogen (females who have anorexia)
- Decreased testosterone (males who have anorexia)

STANDARDIZED SCREENING TOOLS ⊙EBP
- Eating Disorder Inventory
- Eating Disorder Examination
- Eating Attitudes Test

PATIENT-CENTERED CARE

NURSING CARE

- Perform self-assessment regarding possible feelings of frustration regarding the client's eating behaviors, the belief that the disorder is self-imposed, or the need to nurture rather than care for the client.
- Provide a highly structured milieu in an acute care unit for the client requiring intensive therapy.
- Develop and maintain a trusting nurse/ client relationship through consistency and therapeutic communication.
- Use a positive approach and support to promote client self-esteem and positive self-image.
- Encourage client decision-making and participation in the plan of care to allow for a sense of control.
- Establish realistic goals for weight loss or gain.
- Promote cognitive-behavioral therapies. ⊙EBP
  - Cognitive reframing
  - Relaxation techniques
  - Journal writing
  - Desensitization exercises
- Monitor vital signs, intake and output, and weight (2 to 3 lb/week is medically acceptable).
- Use behavioral contracts to modify client behaviors.
- Reward the client for positive behaviors (completing meals or consuming a set number of calories).
- Closely monitor the client during and after meals to prevent purging, which can necessitate accompanying the client to the bathroom.
- Monitor the client for maintenance of appropriate exercise.
- Encourage self-care activities.
- Incorporate the family when appropriate in client education and discharge planning.

- Work with a dietitian to provide nutrition education to include correcting misinformation regarding food, meal planning, and food selection. ⊙TC
  - Consider the client's preferences and ability to consume food when developing the initial eating plan.
  - A structured and inflexible eating schedule at the start of therapy, only permitting food during scheduled times, promotes new eating habits and discourages binge or binge-purge behavior.
  - Provide small, frequent meals, which are better tolerated and will help prevent the client from feeling overwhelmed.
  - Provide liquid supplement as prescribed.
  - Provide a diet high in fiber to prevent constipation.
  - Provide a diet low in sodium to prevent fluid retention.
  - Limit high-fat and gassy foods during the start of treatment.
  - Administer a multivitamin and mineral supplement.
  - Instruct the client to avoid caffeine to reduce the risk for increased energy, resulting in difficulty controlling eating disorder behaviors. Caffeine also can be used by clients as a substitute for healthy eating.
- Make arrangements for the client to attend individual, group, and family therapy to assist in resolving personal issues contributing to the eating disorder.

MEDICATIONS

Selective serotonin reuptake inhibitors

Fluoxetine

NURSING ACTIONS
- Instruct the client that medication can take 1 to 3 weeks for initial response, with up to 2 months for maximal response.
- Instruct the client to avoid hazardous activities (driving, operating heavy equipment/machinery) until individual adverse effects are known.
- Instruct the client to notify the provider if sexual dysfunction occurs and is intolerable.

INTERPROFESSIONAL CARE

- A registered dietitian should be involved to provide the client with nutritional and dietary guidance. ⊙TC
- Consistency of care among all staff is important.

CLIENT EDUCATION

CARE AFTER DISCHARGE
- Assist the client to develop and implement a maintenance plan related to weight management.
- Encourage follow-up treatment in an outpatient setting.
- Encourage client participation in a support group.
- Continue individual and family therapy as indicated.

COMPLICATIONS

Refeeding syndrome

Refeeding syndrome is the potentially fatal complication that can occur when fluids, electrolytes, and carbohydrates are introduced to a severely malnourished client.

NURSING ACTIONS
- Care for the client in a hospital setting.
- Consult with the provider and dietitian to develop a controlled rate of nutritional support during initial treatment. Q_{TC}
- Monitor blood electrolytes, and administer fluid replacement as prescribed.

Cardiac dysrhythmias, severe bradycardia, and hypotension

NURSING ACTIONS
- Place the client on continuous cardiac monitoring.
- Monitor vital signs frequently.
- Report changes in the client's status to the provider.

Active Learning Scenario

A nurse is caring for a client who has anorexia nervosa of the restricting type. The client refuses to eat and exhibits severe anxiety when food is offered. The nurse plans to use desensitization as a behavioral therapy. Use the ATI Active Learning Template: Therapeutic Procedure to complete this item.

DESCRIPTION OF PROCEDURE

INDICATIONS

OUTCOMES/EVALUATION

NURSING INTERVENTIONS: Identify at least two.

Case Study Exercises Key

1. **ANOREXIA NERVOSA:** B, D, F;
   BULIMIA NERVOSA: A, C, E, G

   When taking action, the nurse should identify amenorrhea, fear of gaining weight, and severe dieting are findings associated with anorexia nervosa. Dental erosion, loss of bone density, esophageal tears, and menstrual irregularities are findings associated with bulimia nervosa.

   Ⓝ *NCLEX® Connection: Psychosocial Integrity, Mental Health Concepts*

2. A, C, D, E. **CORRECT:** The nurse should identify that hypokalemia, hyponatremia, hypochloremia, and hypophosphatemia are electrolyte imbalances associated with anorexia nervosa.

   Ⓝ *NCLEX® Connection: Reduction of Risk Potential, Laboratory Values*

Application Exercises

1. A nurse is obtaining a nursing history from a client who has a new diagnosis of anorexia nervosa. Which of the following questions should the nurse include? (Select all that apply.)
   A. "What is your relationship like with your family?"
   B. "Why do you want to lose weight?"
   C. "Would you describe your current eating habits?"
   D. "At what weight do you believe you will look better?"
   E. "Can you discuss your feelings about your appearance?"

2. A nurse is caring for an adolescent client who has anorexia nervosa with recent rapid weight loss and a current weight of 90 lb. Which of the following statements indicates the client is experiencing the cognitive distortion of catastrophizing?
   A. "Life isn't worth living if I gain weight."
   B. "Don't pretend like you don't know how fat I am."
   C. "If I could be skinny, I know I'd be popular."
   D. "When I look in the mirror, I see myself as obese."

3. A nurse is caring for a client who has bulimia nervosa with purging behavior. Which of the following is an expected finding? (Select all that apply.)
   A. Amenorrhea
   B. Hypokalemia
   C. Yellowing of the skin
   D. Slightly elevated body weight
   E. Presence of lanugo on the face

4. A nurse is contributing to the plan of care for a client who has anorexia nervosa with binge-eating and purging behavior. Which of the following interventions should the nurse include?
   A. Allow the client to select preferred meal times.
   B. Establish consequences for purging behavior.
   C. Provide the client with a high-fat diet at the start of treatment.
   D. Implement one-to-one observation during meal times.

5. A nurse is caring for a client who has bulimia nervosa and has stopped purging behavior. The client tells the nurse about fears of gaining weight. Which of the following responses should the nurse make?
   A. "Many clients are concerned about their weight. However, the dietitian will ensure that you don't get too many calories in your diet."
   B. "Instead of worrying about your weight, try to focus on other problems at this time."
   C. "I understand you have concerns about your weight, but first, let's talk about your recent accomplishments."
   D. "You are not overweight, and the staff will ensure that you do not gain weight while you are in the hospital. We know that is important to you."

Active Learning Scenario Key

Using the ATI Active Learning Template: Therapeutic Procedure

DESCRIPTION OF PROCEDURE: Systematic desensitization is the planned, progressive, or graduated exposure to anxiety-provoking stimuli. During exposure, the anxiety response is suppressed through the use of relaxation techniques.

INDICATIONS: Systematic desensitization is appropriate for clients who have anorexia nervosa and anxiety related to food and eating.

OUTCOMES/EVALUATION: The client will effectively use relaxation techniques to suppress the anxiety response during meal times.

NURSING INTERVENTIONS
- Reinforce to the client relaxation techniques.
- Gradually expose the client to food, starting with small amounts of a food.
- Stay with the client during meals to assist with relaxation.
- Reward the client for food intake.
- Use a positive approach to communicate the procedure and expectations to the client.

(N) *NCLEX® Connection: Psychosocial Integrity, Behavioral Management*

Application Exercises Key

1. **A, C, E. CORRECT:** A nursing history of a client who has anorexia nervosa should include an assessment of family and interpersonal relationships, current eating habits, and the client's perception of the issue. Asking a "why" question promotes a defensive client response and is therefore nontherapeutic. Questions that promote cognitive distortion place the focus on weight and imply that the client's current appearance is not acceptable.

(N) *NCLEX® Connection: Psychosocial Integrity, Mental Health Concepts*

2. **A. CORRECT:** This statement reflects the cognitive distortion of catastrophizing because the client's perception of their appearance or situation is much worse than their current condition. The other statements reflect the cognitive distortion of personalization, overgeneralization, and a perception of distorted body image.

(N) *NCLEX® Connection: Psychosocial Integrity, Mental Health Concepts*

3. **B, D. CORRECT:** Hypokalemia is an expected finding of purging-type bulimia nervosa. Most clients who have bulimia nervosa maintain a weight within a normal range or slightly higher. Amenorrhea is an expected finding of anorexia nervosa rather than bulimia nervosa. Yellowing of the skin is an expected finding in anorexia nervosa rather than bulimia nervosa. Lanugo is an expected finding of anorexia nervosa rather than bulimia nervosa.

(N) *NCLEX® Connection: Psychosocial Integrity, Mental Health Concepts*

4. **D. CORRECT:** Closely monitor the client during and after meals to prevent purging. Provide a highly structured milieu, including meal times, for the client requiring acute care for the treatment of anorexia nervosa. Use a positive approach to client care that includes rewards rather than consequences. Limit high-fat and gas-producing foods at the start of treatment.

(N) *NCLEX® Connection: Psychosocial Integrity, Behavioral Management*

5. **C. CORRECT:** The correct statement acknowledges the client's concern and then focuses the conversation on the client's accomplishments, which can promote client self-esteem and self-image. Statements that minimize and generalize the client's concern are nontherapeutic responses.

(N) *NCLEX® Connection: Psychosocial Integrity, Mental Health Concepts*

CHAPTER 20 **Somatic Symptom and Related Disorders**

Clients who have somatic symptom and related disorders are often encountered in primary care settings. It is important that nurses are familiar with these disorders, as well as their role when caring for these clients. Somatic symptom and related disorders include somatic symptom disorder, illness anxiety disorder, functional neurological symptom disorder, factitious disorder, and psychological factors affecting other medical conditions.

Somatic symptom disorder

Somatization is the expression of psychological stress through physical symptoms. The physical manifestations of somatic symptom disorder cannot be explained by underlying pathology.

- Somatic symptoms cause distress for clients and often lead to long-term use of health care services. Symptoms can be vague or exaggerated. The course of the disease can be acute but is often chronic, with periods of remission and exacerbation.
- Clients who have somatic symptom disorder spend a significant amount of time worrying about their physical symptoms to the point where it assumes a central role in the client's life and relationships. Clients often reject a psychological diagnosis as the cause for their physical symptoms. They seek care from several providers, increasing medical costs.
- Clients are usually seen initially in a primary or medical care setting rather than a mental health setting.
- Anxiety and depression are often comorbidities.

DATA COLLECTION

RISK FACTORS

- First-degree relative who has somatic symptom disorder
- Decreased levels of neurotransmitters: serotonin and endorphins
- Depressive disorder, personality disorder, or anxiety disorder
- Low socioeconomic status
- Adverse childhood experiences
- Learned helplessness

EXPECTED FINDINGS

- Somatic symptoms that disrupt the client's daily life
- Excessive preoccupation with somatic symptoms
- Increased level of anxiety about somatic symptoms
- Somatic symptoms are usually present (though actual symptoms can vary) for longer than 6 months.
- Remissions and exacerbations of somatic symptoms
- Probable alcohol or other substance use
- Client overmedication with analgesics and antianxiety medications
- High utilization of health services and multiple health care providers

LABORATORY AND DIAGNOSTIC TESTS

CT scans and MRIs can be performed to rule out underlying pathology.

DATA COLLECTION TOOLS

Patient Health Questionnaire 15 (PHQ-15): Used to identify the presence of the 15 most commonly reported somatic symptoms Q EBP

- Abdominal pain
- Back pain
- Pain in the extremities/joints
- Menstrual problems or cramps
- Headaches
- Chest pain
- Dizziness
- Fainting
- Heart pounding or racing
- Dyspnea
- Problems or pain with sexual intercourse
- Problems with bowel elimination (constipation/diarrhea)
- Nausea, indigestion, or gas
- Lethargy
- Problems sleeping

PATIENT-CENTERED CARE

NURSING CARE

- Accept somatic symptoms as being real to the client.
- Monitor for suicidal ideation and thoughts of self-harm.
- Identify the cultural impact on the client's view of health and illness.
- Identify secondary gains from somatic symptoms (attention, distraction from personal obligations or problems).
- Report new physical symptoms to the provider.
- Limit the amount of time allowed to discuss somatic symptoms.
- Encourage independence in self-care.
- Encourage verbalization of feelings.
- Reinforce teaching with the client on alternative coping mechanisms.
- Reinforce teaching with the client on assertiveness techniques.
- Encourage daily physical exercise.

Reattribution treatment

Work with the provider to provide reattribution treatment, which assists clients to identify the link between physical symptoms and psychological factors while promoting a sense of caring and understanding.

FOUR STAGES OF REATTRIBUTION TREATMENT Qᴛᴄ
- **Stage 1: Feeling understood:** Use therapeutic communication, active listening, and empathy to obtain a thorough history of symptoms while focusing on the client's perception of the symptoms and their cause. This stage also includes a brief physical data collection.
- **Stage 2: Broadening the agenda:** Provide acknowledgment of the client's concerns and provide feedback about data collection findings.
- **Stage 3: Making the link:** Use therapeutic communication to acknowledge the lack of a physical cause for the symptoms while allowing the client to maintain self-esteem.
- **Stage 4: Negotiating further treatment:** Work with the provider and client to develop a treatment plan that allows for regular follow-up visits.

MEDICATIONS

Administer medications as prescribed.
- Analgesics
- Antidepressants
- Anxiolytics

CLIENT EDUCATION

- Participate in individual and group therapy.
- Utilize prescribed medications.
- Assist a case manager to develop a follow-up appointment schedule with provider every 4 to 6 weeks. This strategy provides set appointments and decreases the need for unscheduled health care, as well as medical costs associated with laboratory and diagnostic tests if treatment from other providers is preferred. Qᴇʙᴘ

Illness anxiety disorder

Misinterprets physical manifestations as evidence of a serious disease process. Illness anxiety disorder, previously known as hypochondriasis, can lead to obsessive thoughts and fears about illness.
- Clients who have illness anxiety disorder are overly aware of bodily sensations and attribute them to a serious illness. Physical manifestations can be minimal or absent. However, clients still have a preoccupation about having an undiagnosed, serious illness.
- Clients research their suspected disease excessively and examine themselves repeatedly, such as examining throat in the mirror.
- Clients might either seek numerous medical opinions or avoid seeking health care so as not to increase their anxiety.
- Clients continue to have anxiety despite negative diagnostic tests and reassurance from the provider.

DATA COLLECTION

RISK FACTORS

- First-degree relative who has illness anxiety disorder
- Previous losses or disappointments resulting in feelings of anger, guilt, or hostility
- Childhood trauma, maltreatment , or neglect
- Depressive disorder or anxiety disorder
- Major life stressor
- Low self-esteem

EXPECTED FINDINGS

- Excessive anxiety that a serious illness is present or will be acquired. This anxiety is present for more than 6 months, though the actual illness the client fears can change.
- Preoccupation with performance of behaviors that are health-related (performing a daily breast self-exam due to fear of breast cancer).
- Some clients have illness anxiety disorder that is the **health-seeking type** (frequently seeking medical care and diagnostic tests), while others exhibit the **care-avoidant type** (avoids all contact with providers due to the correlation with increased levels of anxiety).

LABORATORY AND DIAGNOSTIC TESTS

CT scans and MRIs can be performed to rule out underlying pathology.

PATIENT-CENTERED CARE

NURSING CARE

- Build rapport and trust with client.
- Encourage independence in self-care.

MEDICATIONS

Administer medications as prescribed.
- Antidepressants
- Anxiolytics

CLIENT EDUCATION

- Participate in individual and group therapy.
- Attend community support groups.
- Utilize prescribed medications.
- Collaborate with the provider to receive brief, frequent office visits.
- Verbalize any feelings.
- Utilize alternative coping mechanisms.
- Perform stress management techniques.

Functional neurological symptom disorder

Functional neurological symptom disorder, previously known as conversion disorder, results when a client exhibits neurologic manifestations in the absence of a neurologic diagnosis. Clients who have functional neurological symptom disorder transmit emotional or psychological stressors into physical manifestations.

- Neurologic manifestations can cause extreme anxiety and distress in some clients, while others can exhibit a lack of emotional concern (la belle indifference).
- The neurologic manifestation causes a significant impairment in multiple aspects of the client's life.
- Clients who have functional neurological symptom disorder have deficits in voluntary motor or sensory functions (blindness, paralysis, seizures, gait disorders, hearing loss).

DATA COLLECTION

RISK FACTORS

- First-degree relative who has functional neurological symptom disorder
- Childhood physical or sexual abuse
- Comorbid psychiatric conditions
  - Depressive disorder
  - Anxiety disorder
  - Posttraumatic stress disorder
  - Personality disorder
  - Other somatic disorder
- Comorbid medical or neurologic condition
- Recent acute stressful event
- Female sex
- Adolescent or young adult
- Low socioeconomic status, low educational status

EXPECTED FINDINGS

- Manifestations of an alteration in voluntary motor or sensory function
  - Motor: Paralysis, movement/gait disorders, seizure-like movements
  - Sensory: Blindness, inability to speak (aphonia), inability to smell (anosmia), numbness, deafness, tingling/burning sensations
- Clients who have an extreme desire to become pregnant can manifest a false pregnancy (pseudocyesis).

LABORATORY AND DIAGNOSTIC TESTS

CT scans and MRIs can be performed to rule out underlying pathology.

PATIENT-CENTERED CARE

NURSING CARE

- Build rapport and trust with clients.
- Ensure safety of clients.
- Encourage verbalization of feelings. Assist the client to identify the psychological trigger of the manifestation. For example, a client's sudden blindness can be a functional neurological symptom manifestation in response to seeing their partner being intimate with someone else.
- Instruct client on alternative coping mechanisms.
- Instruct client on stress management techniques.
- Understand the incidence of remissions and recurrence. Remission occurs without intervention in approximately 95% of clients, especially if the onset of manifestations is due to an acute stressful event.
  - Relapse rate is approximately 20% usually within 1 year of initial diagnosis.

MEDICATIONS

Administer medications as prescribed.
- Antidepressants
- Anxiolytics

CLIENT EDUCATION

- Participate in individual and group therapy.
- Attend community support groups.
- Utilize prescribed medications.

Psychological factors affecting other medical conditions

Psychological and behavioral factors can play a role in any medical condition. The mind-body connection has been the subject of research, proving a link between a client's psychological state and their physical condition.

- The development of certain medical conditions (heart disease, cancer) has been linked to clients who have depressive and anxiety disorders.
- Other medical conditions have been found to be caused or perpetuated by a psychological or behavioral factor.

DATA COLLECTION

RISK FACTORS

- Chronic stressors
- Depressive disorder or anxiety disorder
- Malfunction of neurotransmitters

EXPECTED FINDINGS

- A confirmed medical diagnosis
- A psychological or behavioral factor that is linked to the medical diagnosis in one of the following ways
  - Contributes to the development, exacerbation, or delayed recovery of the medical diagnosis
  - Interferes with the client's adherence to the treatment of the medical diagnosis
  - Places the client at increased risk for physical health problems
  - Causes or exacerbates physical manifestations or the client's need for medical treatment

PATIENT-CENTERED CARE

NURSING CARE

- Discuss the client's physical exam findings.
- Monitor for suicidal ideation, and thoughts of self-harm. Qs
- Explore the client's feelings and fears.
- Allow the client time to express feelings.
- Instruct the client on alternative coping mechanisms.
- Instruct the client on assertiveness techniques.
- Address both physical and psychological needs.
- Administer prescribed medications.
- Provide care that meets both the physical and psychological needs of the client.

CLIENT EDUCATION

- Participate in treatment plan.
- Utilize prescribed medications.

Factitious disorder

- Factitious disorder (previously known as Munchausen syndrome) is the conscious decision by the client to report physical or psychological manifestations. The falsification of manifestations is done in the absence of personal gain by the client other than possible fulfillment of an emotional need for attention. In some cases, clients inflict self-injury.
- **Factitious disorder imposed on another** (previously known as Munchausen syndrome by proxy) is present when the client deliberately causes injury or illness to a vulnerable person. The emotional need for attention or relief of responsibility remains a possible motivating factor.
- Clients often have an average or above-average IQ. The client is dramatic in the description of the illness, uses proper medical terminology, and is often hesitant for the provider to speak to family members or prior providers.
- The client often reports new manifestations following negative test results.
- Factitious disorder differs from malingering. Factitious disorder is a mental illness, while malingering is not. Malingering is consciously motivated and driven by personal gain (disability benefits, evasion of military service, etc.).

DATA COLLECTION

RISK FACTORS

- History of emotional or physical distress, child maltreatment, or frequent/chronic childhood illnesses requiring hospitalizations
- Impaired neurologic ability for information processing
- Dependent personality
- Borderline personality disorder

EXPECTED FINDINGS

- Report of false physical and psychological manifestations
- Possible evidence of self-injury (factitious disorder) or injury to others (factitious disorder imposed on another)

LABORATORY AND DIAGNOSTIC TESTS

CT scans and MRIs can be performed to rule out underlying pathology.

PATIENT-CENTERED CARE

NURSING CARE

- Perform a self-assessment prior to care.
- Avoid confrontation.
- Build rapport and trust with client.
- Ensure safety of client and vulnerable persons affected by the client.
- Instruct client on alternative coping mechanisms.
- Instruct client on stress management techniques.
- Communicate openly with the health care team any suspicions of factitious disorder or factitious disorder imposed on another. This action can help reduce medical costs and possible unnecessary treatments/ surgical procedures. Qᴛᴄ

CLIENT EDUCATION

- Participate in individual and group therapy.
- Attend community support groups.
- Utilize prescribed medications.
- Verbalize any feelings.

Application Exercises

1. A nurse is discussing the risk factors for somatic symptom disorder with a newly licensed nurse. Which of the following risk factors should the nurse include? (Select all that apply.)

   A. Age older than 65 years

   B. Anxiety disorder

   C. Childhood trauma

   D. Coronary artery disease

   E. Obesity

2. A nurse is reviewing the medical record of a client who has functional neurological symptom disorder. Which of the following findings should the nurse identify as placing the client at risk for functional neurological symptom disorder?

   A. Death of a child 2 months ago

   B. Recent weight loss of 30 lb

   C. Retirement 1 year ago

   D. History of migraine headaches

3. A nurse is collecting data for a client who has illness anxiety disorder. Which of the following findings are expected for this disorder? (Select all that apply.)

   A. Obsessive thoughts about disease

   B. History of childhood maltreatment

   C. Avoidance of health care providers

   D. Depressive disorder

   E. Narcissistic personality

4. A nurse is assisting with developing a plan of care for a client who has functional neurological symptom disorder. Which of the following actions should the nurse include?

   A. Encourage the client to spend time alone in their room.

   B. Monitor the client for self-harm once per day.

   C. Allow the client unlimited time to discuss physical manifestations.

   D. Discuss alternative coping strategies with the client.

5. A nurse is caring for several clients. Which of the following client statements should the nurse identify as expected for factitious disorder imposed on another?

   A. "I had to pretend I was injured in order to get disability benefits."

   B. "I know that my abdominal pain is caused by a malignant tumor."

   C. "I needed to make my child sick so that someone else would take care of them for a while."

   D. "I became deaf when I heard that my partner was having an affair with my best friend."

Active Learning Scenario

A nurse is caring for a client who has psychological factors affecting other medical conditions.
Use the ATI Active Learning Template: System Disorder to complete the following.

EXPECTED FINDINGS: Identify at least two.

RISK FACTORS: Identify the risk factors of psychological factors affecting other medical conditions.

NURSING CARE: Identify at least three nursing interventions for this client.

Active Learning Scenario Key

Using the ATI Active Learning Template: System Disorder

EXPECTED FINDINGS

- A psychological or behavioral factor that is linked to a medical diagnosis in one of the following ways
  - Contributes to the development or exacerbation of the medical diagnosis
  - Interferes with the client's adherence to the treatment of the medical diagnosis
  - Places the client at increased risk for physical health problems and delays recovery
  - Causes or exacerbates physical manifestations or the client's need for medical treatment

RISK FACTORS: Chronic stressors, depressive disorder or anxiety disorder, and imbalance of neurotransmitters

NURSING CARE

- Discuss physical data collection findings with client.
- Monitor for suicidal ideation and thoughts of self-harm.
- Explore the client's feelings and fears.
- Allow the client time to express feelings.
- Instruct the client on alternative coping mechanisms.
- Instruct the client on assertiveness techniques.
- Address both physical and psychological needs.
- Administer prescribed medications.

Ⓝ *NCLEX® Connection: Psychosocial Integrity, Mental Health Concepts*

Application Exercises Key

1. B, C. **CORRECT:** When taking action and discussing risk factors for somatic symptom disorder with a newly licensed nurse, the nurse should include the following. Anxiety disorder and childhood trauma are risk factors for somatic symptom disorder. Age 16 to 25 years is a risk factor for somatic symptom disorder. Coronary artery disease and obesity are not risk factors for somatic symptom disorder.

   Ⓝ *NCLEX® Connection: Health Promotion and Maintenance, Health Promotion/Disease Prevention*

2. A. **CORRECT:** When taking action and reviewing the medical record of a client who has functional neurological symptom disorder, the nurse should identify the following as risk factors. The death of a child 2 months ago is an acute stressor that places the client at risk for functional neurological symptom disorder. A recent weight loss of 30 lb does not place the client at risk for functional neurological symptom disorder. Recent acute stress can be a risk factor. Retiring 1 year ago does not place the client at risk for functional neurological symptom disorder. PTSD can be a risk factor. A history of migraine headaches does not place the client at risk for functional neurological symptom disorder. History of depression can be a risk factor.

   Ⓝ *NCLEX® Connection: Health Promotion and Maintenance, Health Promotion/Disease Prevention*

3. A, B, C, D. **CORRECT:** When collecting data for a client who has illness anxiety disorder, the nurse should expect the following findings. Obsessive thoughts about disease is an expected finding in a client who has illness anxiety disorder. A history of childhood maltreatment is an expected finding in a client who has illness anxiety disorder. Avoidance of health care providers is an expected finding in clients who have illness anxiety disorder of the care-avoidant type. A depressive disorder is an expected finding in a client who has illness anxiety disorder. Low self-esteem is an expected finding in a client who has illness anxiety disorder.

   Ⓝ *NCLEX® Connection: Psychosocial Integrity, Mental Health Concepts*

4. D. **CORRECT:** When assisting with developing a plan of care for the client who has functional neurological symptom disorder, the nurse should discuss alternative coping strategies with the client. The nurse should encourage the client to communicate with others and participate in group therapy and support, continuously monitor the client for risk of self-harm, and establish a time limit for discussion of physical manifestations.

   Ⓝ *NCLEX® Connection: Psychosocial Integrity, Mental Health Concepts*

5. C. **CORRECT:** A client who has factitious disorder imposed on another often consciously injures another person or causes them to be sick due to a personal need for attention or relief of responsibility. A client's falsification of an illness or injury for the purpose of personal gain is malingering. Although clients who have factitious disorder often use proper medical terminology, a client's fear of a serious illness is expected with illness anxiety disorder. Developing a sensory impairment due to an acute stressor is an expected finding of functional neurological symptom disorder.

   Ⓝ *NCLEX® Connection: Psychosocial Integrity, Mental Health Concepts*

NCLEX® Connections

When reviewing the following chapters, keep in mind the relevant topics and tasks of the NCLEX outline.

Health Promotion and Maintenance

HIGH-RISK BEHAVIORS: Provide information for prevention of high-risk behaviors.

Psychosocial Integrity

GRIEF AND LOSS
Identify client reaction to loss.

Provide client with resources to adjust to loss/bereavement.

MENTAL HEALTH CONCEPTS
Recognize a change in the client's mental status.

Explore reasons for client noncompliance with treatment plan.

Identify client symptoms of acute or chronic mental illness.

UNIT 4   SPECIFIC POPULATIONS

CHAPTER 21   *Care of Clients Who Are Dying and/or Grieving*

Clients experience loss in many aspects of their lives. Grief is the inner emotional response to loss and is exhibited in as many ways as there are individuals.

Bereavement includes both grief and mourning (the outward display of loss) as a person deals with the death of a significant individual. Bereavement can result in depression. A bereavement exclusion was previously used when a client experienced manifestations of depression within the first 2 months after a significant loss. Now, a client can receive a diagnosis of depression during this time so that needed treatment is not delayed.

End-of-life care is an important aspect of nursing care that attempts to meet the client's physical and psychosocial needs. End-of-life issues include decision-making in a highly stressful time during which the nurse must consider the desires of the client and the family. End-of-life care can include palliative interventions which promote comfort. Qᴘᴄᴄ

Communicate treatment decision with other health care personnel for a smooth transition during this time of stress, grief, and bereavement.

TYPES OF LOSS

Necessary loss: Part of the cycle of life; anticipated, but can still be intensely felt

Actual loss: Any loss of a valued person or item

Perceived loss: Any loss defined by a client that is not obvious to others

Maturational loss: Losses normally expected due to the developmental processes of life

Situational loss: Unanticipated loss caused by an external event

THEORIES OF GRIEF

The mental health care nurse should be aware of the various theories of grief. Though multiple theories are present, they each tend to identify the same underlying feelings that the client who is grieving experiences. Clients might not always experience the stages or tasks in the same order, and the length of time required to progress through grief will vary. Qᴇʙᴘ

Kübler-Ross: Five stages of grief

Denial: The client has difficulty believing a terminal diagnosis or loss.

Anger: Anger is directed toward self, others, or objects.

Bargaining: The client negotiates for more time or a cure.

Depression: The client is overwhelmingly saddened by the inability to change the situation.

Acceptance: The client accepts what is happening and plans for the future.

Bowlby: Four stages of grief

Identifies behaviors that are observed in clients who are grieving. These stages are present in clients as young as 6 months of age.

Numbness or protest: The client is in denial over the reality of the loss and experiences feelings of shock.

Disequilibrium: The client focuses on the loss and has an intense desire to regain what was lost.

Disorganization and despair: The client feels hopelessness, which impacts the client's ability to carry out tasks of daily living.

Reorganization: The client reaches acceptance of the loss.

Engel: Five stages of grief

Shock and disbelief: The client experiences a sense of numbness and denial over the loss.

Developing awareness: The client becomes aware of the reality of the loss, resulting in intense feelings of grief. This begins within hours of the loss.

Restitution: The client carries out cultural/religious rituals (a funeral) following the loss.

Resolution of the loss: The client is preoccupied with the loss. Over about a 12-month time period, this preoccupation gradually decreases.

Recovery: The client moves past the preoccupation and forward with life.

Worden: Four tasks of mourning

Completion of four active tasks empowering the mourner to resolve grief

Task I: Accepting the reality of the loss

Task II: Processing the pain of grief. The client uses coping mechanisms to deal with the emotional pain of the loss.

Task III: Adjusting to a world without the lost entity. The client changes the environment to accommodate the absence of the deceased.

Task IV: Finding an enduring connection with the lost entity in the midst of embarking on a new life. The client finds a way to keep the lost entity a part of their life while at the same time moving forward with life and establishing new relationships.

CONCEPT OF DEATH AND GRIEF ACROSS THE LIFESPAN

Infant and toddler

- Increased crying and irritability
- Looking for the person who has died
- Regression

Preschoolers

- Do not understand that "dead" is not "alive"
- Repetitive questions
- Regression

School-age

- Developing an understanding of irreversibility of death
- Play used to recreate death event
- Mood lability

Adolescents

- Conceptualize and understand death
- Sudden abnormal behaviors
- Increase in risk-taking behaviors
- Depression or thoughts of self-harm

FACTORS INFLUENCING LOSS, GRIEF, AND COPING ABILITY

- Current stage of development
- Interpersonal relationships and social support network
- Type and significance of the loss
- Culture and ethnicity
- Spiritual and religious beliefs and practices
- Prior experience with loss
- Socioeconomic status

RISK FACTORS FOR COMPLICATED GRIEVING

- Being dependent upon the deceased
- Unexpected death at a young age, through violence, or by a socially unacceptable manner
- Inadequate coping skills or lack of social support
- Preexisting mental health issues (depression, substance use disorder)

PROTECTIVE FACTORS

- Regular spiritual or religious practices
- A well-developed sense of personal well-being
- A sense of financial control
- No additional or concurrent losses

NURSING ACTIONS

- Clients who are experiencing a complicated grief response commonly experience a loss of self-esteem and a sense of worthlessness not associated with normal grief.
- Check the client for risk factors, and identify a normal versus a complicated grief response.

DATA COLLECTION

Normal grief

- This grief is considered uncomplicated.
- Emotions can include anger, resentment, withdrawal, hopelessness, and guilt but should change to acceptance with time.
- Client should achieve some acceptance by 6 months after the loss.
- Somatic manifestations can include chest pain, palpitations, headaches, nausea, changes in sleep patterns, or fatigue.
- The nurse should collect data from the client to identify a normal vs. complicated grief response.

Anticipatory grief

- This grief implies the "letting go" of an object or person before the loss, as in the case of a terminal illness.
- Individuals have the opportunity to grieve before the actual loss.

Prolonged grief disorder

- Persistent, prolonged, severe grief that is manifested by identity confusion and separation distress.
- Comorbidities include cardiac disease, depression, anxiety, substance use, immunological deficiency, and reduced quality of life.
- Intense yearning for the deceased person
- Increased risk for suicide

Complicated grief

Delayed or inhibited grief
- The client does not demonstrate the expected behaviors of the normal grief process.
- Cultural expectations can influence the development of delayed or inhibited grief.
- Clients can remain in the denial stage of grief for an extended period of time.
- Due to client's inability to progress through the stages/tasks of grief, a subsequent minor loss (even years later) can trigger the grief response.

Distorted or exaggerated grief response

- Experiences the feelings and somatic manifestations associated with normal grief but to an exaggerated level.
- Unable to perform activities of daily living
- Can remain in the anger stage of the grief process and can direct the anger towards themselves or others
- Can develop clinical depression

Chronic or prolonged grief

- This maladaptive response is difficult to identify due to the varying lengths of time required by clients to work through the stages/tasks of grief.
- Clients can remain in the denial stage of grief and remain unable to accept the reality of the loss.
- Chronic or prolonged grief can result in the client's inability to perform activities of daily living.

Disenfranchised grief: This grief entails an experienced loss that cannot be publicly shared or is not socially accepted (suicide and abortion).

NURSING INTERVENTIONS

Facilitating mourning

- Allow time for the grieving process.
- Educate the client and family on the stages and tasks associated with the grieving process.
- Identify expected grieving behaviors, (crying, somatic manifestations, anxiety).
- Use therapeutic communication. Name the emotion that the client is feeling. For example, a nurse might say, "You sound as though you are angry. Anger is a normal feeling for someone who has lost a loved one. Tell me about how you are feeling." Qpcc
- Use silence and personal presence to facilitate mourning of feelings.
- Avoid communication that inhibits open expression of feelings (offering false reassurance, giving advice, changing the subject, taking the focus away from the individual who is grieving).
- When relating to someone who is bereaved, avoid clichés ("They are in a better place now."). Rather, encourage the individual to share memories about the deceased.
- Assist the individual to accept the reality of the loss.
- Support the client's efforts to "move on" in the face of the loss.
- Encourage the building of new relationships.
- Provide continuing support. Encourage the support of family and friends.
- Monitor for indications of ineffective coping (refusing to leave home months after a client's partner has died).
- Encourage the client who is grieving to attend a bereavement or grief support group.
- Recommend a referral for psychotherapy for a client who is having a maladaptive grief response. Qtc
- Reinforce information on available community resources.

- Ask the client if contacting a spiritual adviser would be acceptable, or encourage the client to do so.
- Participate in debriefing provided by professional grief or mental health counselors.
- **Bereavement care:** Given by the health care team to persons who are in the process of dying or care postdeath for those who are grieving and their families, which can include any end-of-life care such as hospice or palliative

Psychosocial care

- Use an interprofessional approach.
- Provide care to the client and the family.
- Discuss specific concerns the client and family can have (financial, role changes). Recommend a social services or other referral as needed.
- Use therapeutic communication to develop and maintain a nurse-client relationship.
- Facilitate communication between the client, family, and provider.
- Encourage the client to participate in religious/spiritual practices that bring comfort and strength, if appropriate.
- Assist the client in clarifying personal values to facilitate effective decision-making.
- Encourage the client to use coping mechanisms that have worked in the past.
- Be cautious with what is said in the presence of a client who is unconscious, as it is widely accepted that hearing is the last of the senses that is lost. Qebp
- Use volunteers when appropriate to provide nonmedical care.
- Facilitate the understanding of information regarding disease progression and treatment choices.

Protection against abandonment and isolation

Decrease the fear of dying alone.
- Make presence known by answering call lights in a timely manner and making frequent contact.
- Keep the client informed of procedure/data collection times.
- Allow family members to remain with the client as much as possible.
- Determine where the client is most comfortable (in a room close to the nurses' station).
- If the client chooses to be at home, move the client's bed to a central location in the home rather than an isolated bedroom. Qpcc

Support for the grieving family

- Suggest that family members plan visits in a manner that promotes client rest.
- Ensure that the family receives appropriate information as the treatment plan changes.
- Provide privacy so family members have the opportunity to communicate and express feelings among themselves.
- Determine family members' desire to provide physical care. Provide instruction as necessary.
- Educate the family about physical changes during active dying.
- Allow families to express feelings.

Active Learning Scenario

A nurse is caring for a client who is dying. Use the ATI Active Learning Template: Basic Concept to complete this item.

UNDERLYING PRINCIPLES
- Define anticipatory grief.
- Identify at least four interventions to provide psychosocial care to the client who is dying.

NURSING INTERVENTIONS: Identify at least two interventions to prevent these feeling of abandonment and isolation in the client who is dying.

Application Exercises

1. A nurse is caring for a client following the loss of a partner due to a terminal illness. Identify the sequence of Engel's five stages of grief that the nurse should expect the client to experience. (Sort the stages of grief in order of occurrence. All steps must be used.)

    A. Developing awareness

    B. Restitution

    C. Shock and disbelief

    D. Recovery

    E. Resolution of the loss

2. A charge nurse is reviewing the Kübler-Ross five stages of grief with a group of newly licensed nurses. Which of the following stages should the charge nurse include in the teaching? (Select all that apply.)

    A. Disequilibrium

    B. Denial

    C. Bargaining

    D. Anger

    E. Depression

3. A nurse is working with a client who has recently lost a guardian. The nurse recognizes that which of the following factors influence a client's grief and coping ability? (Select all that apply.)

    A. Interpersonal relationships

    B. Culture

    C. Birth order

    D. Religious beliefs

    E. Prior experience with loss

4. A nurse is discussing normal grief with a client who recently lost a child. Which of the following statements made by the client indicates understanding? (Select all that apply.)

    A. "I may experience feelings of resentment."

    B. "I will probably withdraw from others."

    C. "I can expect to experience changes in sleep."

    D. "It is possible that I will experience suicidal thoughts."

    E. "It is expected that I will have a loss of self-esteem."

5. A nurse is caring for a client who lost a guardian to cancer last month. The client states, "I'd still have my guardian if the doctor would have made a diagnosis sooner." Which of the following responses should the nurse make?

    A. "You sound angry. Anger is a normal feeling associated with loss."

    B. "I think you would feel better if you talked about your feelings with a support group."

    C. "I understand just how you feel. I felt the same when my guardian died."

    D. "Do other members of your family also feel this way?"

Application Exercises Key

1. C, A, B, E, D

   Step 1: Shock and disbelief is the first stage in Engel's five stages of grief. In this stage, the client experiences a sense of numbness and denial over the loss. Step 2: Developing awareness is the second stage in Engel's five stages of grief. In this stage, the client becomes aware of the reality of the loss, resulting in intense feelings of grief. This begins within hours of the loss. Step 3: Restitution is the third stage in Engel's five stages of grief. In this stage, the client carries out cultural/religious rituals (a funeral) following the loss. Step 4: Resolution of the loss is the fourth stage in Engel's five stages of grief. In this stage, the client is preoccupied with the loss. This preoccupation gradually decreases over about a 12-month time period. Step 5: Recovery is the fifth and final stage in Engel's five stages of grief. In this stage, the client moves past the preoccupation with the loss and moves forward with life.

   Ⓝ *NCLEX: Psychosocial Integrity, Grief and Loss*

2. B, C, D, E. **CORRECT:** The denial stage is when the client has difficulty believing a terminal diagnosis or loss. This is one of the Kübler-Ross five stages of grief. The bargaining stage is when the client negotiates for more time or a cure. This is one of the Kübler-Ross five stages of grief. The anger stage is when the client directs anger toward self, others, or objects. This is one of the Kübler-Ross five stages of grief. The depression stage is when the client mourns and directly confronts feelings related to the loss. This is one of the Kübler-Ross five stages of grief. Disequilibrium is the second stage of Bowlby's four stages of grief.

   Ⓝ *NCLEX® Connection: Psychosocial Integrity, Grief and Loss*

3. A, B, D, E. **CORRECT:** The client's interpersonal relationships are factors that influence the client's reaction to grief and ability to cope. The client's culture is a factor that influences the client's reaction to grief and ability to cope. The client's religious beliefs are factors that influence the client's reaction to grief and ability to cope. The client's prior experience with loss is a factor that influences the client's reaction to grief and ability to cope. Birth order is not a factor that influences grief and ability to cope.

   Ⓝ *NCLEX® Connection: Psychosocial Integrity, Religious and Spiritual Influences on Health*

4. A, B, C. **CORRECT:** Resentment is an emotion that can be associated with normal grief. Withdrawal is an emotion that can be seen with normal grief. Somatic manifestations (changes in sleep patterns) can be associated with normal grief. Suicidal ideations are associated with complicated grieving. The client who is experiencing a distorted or exaggerated grief response can direct anger towards themselves. Assess and monitor the client for thoughts of suicide or self-injury. A client who is experiencing a complicated grief response commonly experiences a loss of self-esteem and a sense of worthlessness. These findings are not associated with normal grief.

   Ⓝ *NCLEX® Connection: Psychosocial Integrity, Therapeutic Communication*

5. A. **CORRECT:** This is a therapeutic response for the nurse to make. This response acknowledges the client's emotion and provides education on the normal grief response. Offering advice is a nontherapeutic communication technique. Minimizing the client's feelings is a nontherapeutic communication technique. Taking the focus away from the client is a nontherapeutic communication technique.

   Ⓝ *NCLEX® Connection: Psychosocial Integrity, Therapeutic Communication*

Active Learning Scenario Key

Using the ATI Active Learning Template: Basic Concept

UNDERLYING PRINCIPLES

- Anticipatory grief allows the client to work through the grieving process and ideally achieve acceptance prior to their actual death. The client's family can also experience anticipatory grief in preparation for their loss.
- Psychosocial care
  - Use an interprofessional approach.
  - Discuss specific concerns the client and family may have (financial, role changes). Recommend a social services or other referral as needed.
  - Use therapeutic communication to develop and maintain a nurse-client relationship.
  - Facilitate communication between the client, family, and provider.
  - Encourage the client to participate in religious/spiritual practices that bring comfort and strength, if appropriate.
  - Assist the client in clarifying personal values to facilitate effective decision-making.
  - Encourage the client to use coping mechanisms that have worked in the past.
  - Be cautious with what is said in the presence of a client who is unconscious, as it is widely accepted that hearing is the last of the senses that is lost.

NURSING INTERVENTIONS

- Make presence known by answering call lights in a timely manner and making frequent contact.
- Keep the client informed of procedure/data collection times.
- Allow family members to remain with the client as much as possible.
- Determine where the client is most comfortable (in a room close to the nurses' station).
- If the client chooses to be at home, move the client's bed to a central location in the home rather than an isolated bedroom.

Ⓝ *NCLEX® Connection: Psychosocial Integrity, Grief and Loss*

CHAPTER 22

CHAPTER 22 *Mental Health Issues of Children and Adolescents*

Childhood and adolescent mental health and neurodevelopment disorders are not always easily identified and diagnosed. As a result of this, treatment and interventions can be delayed.

As with adults, children and adolescents may meet the criteria for more than one mental health disorder and have comorbid conditions.

Behaviors displayed by children become problematic when they interfere with home, school, and interactions with peers.

DISORDERS THAT CAN APPEAR DURING CHILDHOOD AND ADOLESCENCE Qs

Depressive disorders, including major depressive disorder and persistent depressive disorder

Anxiety disorders, including separation anxiety disorder and panic disorder

Trauma- and stressor-related disorders, including posttraumatic stress disorder (PTSD)

Substance use disorders, including alcohol use disorder, tobacco use disorder, and cannabis use disorder

Feeding and eating disorders, including anorexia nervosa, bulimia nervosa, and binge eating disorder

Disruptive, impulse control, and conduct disorders, including oppositional defiant disorder, disruptive mood dysregulation disorder, and conduct disorder

Neurodevelopment disorders, including attention deficit/hyperactivity disorder (ADHD), autism spectrum disorder, intellectual development disorder, and specific learning disorder

Bipolar and related disorders

Schizophrenia spectrum and other psychotic disorders

Nonsuicidal self-injury and suicidal behavior disorder; suicide is a leading cause of death for youth between the ages of 10 and 24.

Impulse control disorders, including intermittent explosive disorder

Communication disorders, including stuttering, repetitive language disorder, expressive language disorder, mixed repetitive-expressive disorder and social communication disorder

Tic disorders, including provisional and persistent tic disorder and Tourette's disorder

FACTORS IMPEDING DIAGNOSIS

- Children might not have the language skills and cognitive and emotional development to describe what is happening.
- Children demonstrate a wide variation of "normal" behaviors, especially in different developmental stages.
- It is difficult to determine whether a child's behavior indicates an emotional problem, which can delay diagnosis and interventions.

CHARACTERISTICS OF GOOD MENTAL HEALTH

- Ability to appropriately interpret reality, as well as having a correct perception of the surrounding environment
- Positive self-concept
- Ability to cope with stress and anxiety in an age-appropriate way
- Mastery of developmental tasks
- Ability to express oneself spontaneously and creatively
- Ability to develop and maintain satisfying relationships

DATA COLLECTION

ETIOLOGY AND GENERAL RISK FACTORS

Genetic links or chromosomal abnormalities are associated with some disorders (schizophrenia, bipolar disorder, autism spectrum disorder, ADHD, and intellectual development disorder).

Biochemical: Alterations in neurotransmitters, including norepinephrine, serotonin, or dopamine, contribute to some mental health disorders.

Social and environmental: Severe marital discord, low socioeconomic status, large families, overcrowding, parental criminality, substance use disorders, maternal psychiatric disorders, parental depression, and foster care placement are all risk factors.

Cultural and ethnic: Difficulty with assimilation, potential lack of cultural role models, and potential lack of support from the dominant culture can contribute to mental health issues.

Resiliency: The ability to adapt to changes in the environment, form nurturing relationships, exhibit effective coping strategies, and use problem-solving skills can help an at-risk child avoid the development of a mental health disorder.

Witnessing or experiencing traumatic events (physical or sexual abuse) during the formative years are risk factors.

DEPRESSIVE DISORDERS

RISK FACTORS
- Family history of depression ○EBP
- Physical or sexual abuse or neglect
- Homelessness
- Disputes among parents, conflicts with peers or family, and rejection by peers or family
- Bullying, either as the aggressor or victim, including traditional bullying and cyberbullying behavior
- Engaging in high-risk behaviors
- Learning disabilities
- Chronic illness

EXPECTED FINDINGS
- Feelings of sadness
- Temper tantrums (verbal and behavioral outbursts)
- Loss of appetite
- Nonspecific complaints related to health
- Engaging in solitary play or work
- Changes in appetite, resulting in weight changes
- Changes in sleeping patterns
- Crying
- Loss of energy
- Irritability
- Aggression
- High-risk behavior
- Poor school performance and/or dropping out of school
- Feelings of hopelessness about the future
- Suicidal ideation or suicide attempts

ANXIETY DISORDERS AND TRAUMA- AND STRESSOR-RELATED DISORDERS

EXPECTED FINDINGS
- The anxiety or level of stress interferes with normal growth and development. ○EBP
- The anxiety or level of stress is so serious that the child is unable to function normally at home, in school, and in other areas of life.

Separation anxiety disorder

- This type of disorder is characterized by excessive anxiety when a child is separated from or anticipating separation from home or parents that is developmentally inappropriate. The anxiety can develop into a school phobia or phobia of being left alone. Depression is also common.
- Anxiety can develop after a specific stressor (death of a relative or pet, illness, move, assault).
- Anxiety can progress to a panic disorder or type of phobia.

Posttraumatic stress disorder

- PTSD is precipitated by experiencing, witnessing, or learning of a traumatic event.
- Children and adolescents who have PTSD exhibit psychological indications of anxiety, depression, phobia, or conversion reactions.
- If the anxiety resulting from PTSD is displayed externally, it is often manifested as irritability and aggression with family and friends, poor academic performance, somatic reports, belief that life will be short, and difficulty sleeping.
- Small children can show a decrease in play or engage in play that involves aspects of the traumatic event.

DISRUPTIVE, IMPULSE CONTROL, AND CONDUCT DISORDERS

EXPECTED FINDINGS
- Behavioral problems usually occur in school, home, and social settings. ○EBP
- Comorbid disorders can also be present (ADHD, depression, anxiety, substance use disorders).
- In children and adolescents who have disruptive, impulse control, and conduct disorders, manifestations generally worsen in the following.
  - Situations that require sustained attention (classroom)
  - Unstructured group situations (the playground)

Oppositional defiant disorder

- This disorder is characterized by a recurrent pattern of the following antisocial behaviors.
  - Negativity
  - Disobedience
  - Hostility
  - Defiant behaviors (especially toward authority figures)
  - Stubbornness
  - Argumentativeness
  - Limit testing
  - Unwillingness to compromise
  - Refusal to accept responsibility for misbehavior
- Misbehavior is usually demonstrated at home and directed toward the person best known.
- Children and adolescents who have oppositional defiant disorder do not see themselves as defiant. They view their behavior as a response to unreasonable demands and/or circumstances.
- Children who have this disorder can exhibit low self-esteem, mood lability, and a low frustration threshold.
- Oppositional defiant disorder can develop into conduct disorder.

Disruptive mood dysregulation disorder

- Clients who have this disorder exhibit recurrent temper outbursts that are severe and do not correlate with situation.
  - Temper outbursts are manifested verbally and/or physically and can include aggression.
  - Temper outbursts are not appropriate for the client's developmental level.
- Temper outbursts are present three or more times per week and are observable by others (guardians, peers, teachers) in at least two settings (home, school).
- Mood between the temper outbursts is angry and irritable.
- Onset of this disorder is between the ages of 6 and 18.
- Manifestations are not due to another mental health disorder (bipolar disorder).

Intermittent explosive disorder

Clients who have this disorder exhibit recurrent episodic violent and aggressive behavior with the possibility of hurting people, property, or animals.
- Diagnosed as early as 6 years old (typically between ages 13 to 21 years)
- More males affected
- Includes verbal or physical aggression
- Characterized by aggressive overreaction to normal events, followed by feelings of shame and regret
- Prevents the client's ability to have healthy relationships and/or employment. Can lead to the development of chronic disease (hypertension, diabetes mellitus)

Conduct disorder (childhood or adolescent onset)

- Clients who have conduct disorder demonstrate a persistent pattern of behavior that violates the rights of others or rules and norms of society. Categories of conduct disorder include the following.
  - Aggression to people and animals
  - Destruction of property
  - Deceitfulness or theft
  - Serious violations of rules
- Childhood-onset develops before the age of 10, with males being more prevalent. Adolescent-onset occurs after the age of 10. The ratio of males-to-females is equal in the adolescent stage. Q EBP

CONTRIBUTING FACTORS
- Parental rejection and neglect
- Difficult infant temperament
- Inconsistent child-rearing practices with harsh discipline
- Physical or sexual abuse
- Lack of supervision
- Early institutionalization
- Frequent changing of caregivers
- Large family size
- Association with delinquent peer groups
- Parent with a history of psychological illness
- Chaotic home life
- Lack of male role model

MANIFESTATIONS
- Demonstrates a lack of remorse or care for the feelings of others
- Bullies, threatens, and intimidates others
- Believes that aggression is justified
- Exhibits low self-esteem, irritability, temper outbursts, reckless behavior
- Can demonstrate suicidal ideation
- Can have concurrent learning disorders or impairments in cognitive functioning
- Demonstrates physical cruelty to others and/or animals
- Has used a weapon that could cause serious injuries
- Destroys property of others
- Has run away from home
- Often lies, shoplifts, and is truant from school

NEURODEVELOPMENT DISORDERS

ETIOLOGY AND GENERAL RISK FACTORS
- The prevalence of neurodevelopmental disorders has been increasing in the United States with the current rate of one in six children.
- Change with maturation, and although they typically improve with age, the manifestations and associated problems may persist into adult life.
- Complex and are often the result of more than one factor, as multiple hereditary and environmental influences may affect neurological development

COMORBIDITIES
- Manifestations may present with a variety of other medical conditions.
- Developing an accurate diagnosis can be difficult due to the amount of overlapping manifestations of other conditions.

Attention deficit hyperactivity disorder

Involves the inability of a person to control behaviors requiring sustained attention Q EBP
- Inattention, impulsivity, and hyperactivity are characteristic behaviors of ADHD.
  - **Inattention** is evidenced by a difficulty in paying attention, listening, and focusing.
  - **Hyperactivity** is evidenced by fidgeting, an inability to sit still, running and climbing inappropriately, difficulty with playing quietly, and talking excessively.
  - **Impulsivity** is evidenced by difficulty waiting for turns, constantly interrupting others, and acting without the consideration of consequences.
- Inattentive or impulsive behavior can put the child at risk for injury.
- Behaviors associated with ADHD must be present prior to age 12 and must be present in more than one setting to be diagnosed as ADHD. Behaviors associated with ADHD can receive negative attention from adults and peers.

TYPES OF ADHD
- ADHD predominantly inattentive
- ADHD predominantly hyperactive-impulsive
- Combined type: Client exhibits both inattentive and hyperactive-impulsive behaviors

Autism spectrum disorder

- Autism spectrum disorder is a complex neurodevelopment disorder thought to be of genetic origin with a wide spectrum of behaviors affecting an individual's ability to communicate and interact with others. Cognitive and language development are typically delayed. Characteristic behaviors include inability to maintain eye contact, repetitive actions, and strict observance of routines.
- This type of disorder is present in early childhood and is more common in boys than girls.
- Physical difficulties experienced by the child who has autism spectrum disorder include sensory integration dysfunction, sleep disorders, digestive disorders, feeding disorders, epilepsy, and/or allergies.
- There is a wide variability in functioning. Abilities can range from poor (inability to perform self-care, inability to communicate and relate to others) to high (ability to function at near normal levels).

Intellectual development disorder

- Clients who have intellectual development disorder have an onset of deficits and impairments during the developmental period of infancy or childhood.
- The client has intellectual deficits with mental abilities (reasoning, abstract thinking, academic learning, learning from prior experiences).
- Clients demonstrate impaired ability to maintain personal independence and social responsibility, including activities of daily living, social participation, and the need for ongoing support at school.
- Deficits in the disorder range from mild to severe.

Specific learning disorder

- Client demonstrates persistent difficulty in acquiring reading, writing, or mathematical skills.
- Performance in one or more academic areas is significantly lower than the expected range for the client's age, level of intelligence, or educational level.
- Clients who have specific learning disorder benefit from an individualized education program (IEP).

Communication disorders

- Client demonstrates persistent problems related to language and speech skills.
- Speech dysfluencies, such as stuttering
- Difficulty with conversational skills that are exacerbated by age-related social pressures

PATIENT-CENTERED CARE

NURSING CARE

- Assist with obtaining a complete nursing history to include the following.
  - Mother's pregnancy and birth history
  - Sleeping, eating, and elimination patterns
  - Attachment behaviors
  - Recent weight loss or gain
  - Achievement of developmental milestones
  - Allergies
  - Current medications
  - Peer and family relationships, school performance
  - History of emotional, physical, or sexual abuse
  - Parental perceptions and level of tolerance toward child's behavior
  - Family history, including current members of the household
  - Substance use
    - Tobacco use disorder (cigarettes, cigars, snuff, chewing tobacco)
    - Alcohol, frequency of use, driving under the influence, and family history of alcohol use disorder
    - Illicit drugs or prescription medications to get high, stay calm, lose weight, or stay awake
  - Safety at home and at school
  - Actual or potential risk for self-injury
  - Presence of depression and suicidal ideation, including a plan, the lethality of that plan, and the means to carry out the plan
  - Availability of weapons in the home
- Assist with performing a complete physical examination, including a mental status examination and developmental assessment.
- Use primary prevention (education, peer group discussions, mentoring) to prevent risky behavior and to promote healthy behavior and effective coping.
  - Work with clients to adopt a realistic view of their bodies and to improve overall self-esteem.
  - Identify and reinforce the use of positive coping skills.
  - Employ the use of gun and weapon control strategies.
  - Emphasize the use of seat belts when in motor vehicles.
  - Encourage the use of protective gear for high-impact sports.
  - Reinforce education on contraceptives and other sexual information (transmission and prevention of HIV and other sexually transmitted infections).
  - Encourage abstinence, but keep the lines of communication open to allow the adolescent to discuss sexual practices.
  - Encourage clients and family members to seek professional help if indicated.

- Intervene for clients who have engaged in high-risk behaviors.
  ○ Instruct the client and family on factors that contribute to substance use disorders. Make appropriate referrals when indicated.
  ○ Inform the client and family about support groups in the community for eating disorders, substance use disorders, and general teen support.
  ○ Instruct the client regarding individuals within the school environment and community to whom concerns can be voiced about personal safety and bullying (police officers, school nurses, counselors, teachers).
  ○ Make referrals to social services when indicated.
  ○ Discuss the use and availability of support hotlines.
  ○ Assist with a depression and suicide assessment. Make an immediate referral for professional care when indicated. Qs

INTERVENTIONS

For anxiety disorders
- Providing emotional support that is accepting of regression and other defense mechanisms
- Offering protection during panic levels of anxiety by providing for needs
- Implementing methods to increase client self-esteem and feelings of achievement

For trauma and stressor-related disorders
- Providing assistance with working through traumatic events or losses to reach acceptance
- Encouraging group therapy

For disruptive, impulse control, and conduct disorders and ADHD
- Use a calm, firm, respectful approach with the child.
- Use modeling to show acceptable behavior.
- Obtain the child's attention before giving directions. Provide short and clear explanations.
- Set clear limits on unacceptable behaviors and be consistent.
- Assist with planning physical activities through which the child can use energy and obtain success.
- Assist parents to develop a reward system using methods such as a wall chart or tokens. Encourage the child to participate.
- Focus on the family's and child's strengths, not just the problems.
- Support the parents' efforts to remain hopeful.
- Provide a safe environment for the child and others.
- Provide the child with specific positive feedback when expectations are met.
- Identify issues that result in power struggles.
- Assist the child in developing effective coping mechanisms.
- Encourage the child to participate in group, individual, and family therapy.
- Administer medications (antipsychotics, mood stabilizers, anticonvulsants, antidepressants) and monitor for adverse effects.

For autism spectrum disorder
- Recommend referrals (physical, occupational, and speech therapy) as indicated for early intervention.
- Provide for a structured environment.
- Work with parents to provide consistent and individualized care.
- Encourage parents to participate in the child's care and treatment plan as much as possible.
- Use short, concise, and developmentally appropriate communication.
- Identify desired behaviors and reward them.
- Role-model social skills.
- Role-play situations that involve conflict and conflict resolution strategies.
- Encourage verbal communication.
- Limit self-stimulating and ritualistic behaviors by providing alternative play activities.
- Determine emotional and situational triggers.
- Give plenty of notice before changing routines.
- Carefully monitor the child's behaviors to ensure safety.

For communication disorders
- Rule out autism spectrum disorder.
- Recommend a referral for a hearing test.
- Recommend referrals (occupational and speech therapy) as indicated for early intervention.
- Assist with individualizing interventions and treatment based on the child's specific deficit.
- Work with parents to provide consistent and individualized care.

For tic disorders
- Identify specific behaviors that are associated with the disorder
- Redirect tic behavior.
- Reinforce behavioral therapy techniques (habit reversal and comprehensive behavior intervention therapy [CBIT]).
- Provide protective measures to promote client safety.
- Allow a specific time in which the child is allowed to share feelings related to tic behaviors.
- Encourage parents to participate in the child's care and treatment plan as much as possible.

INTERPROFESSIONAL CARE

- Family therapy enables the client and family to address problems. QEBP
- Cognitive-behavioral therapy is useful to change negative thoughts to positive outcomes when intervening for depressive and disruptive, impulse control, and conduct disorders.
- Grief and trauma intervention (GTI) for children is effective for clients who have a trauma- and stressor-related disorder. GTI encourages narrative expression (drawing, writing, or play) regarding the traumatic event.
- Other therapeutic approaches can include group therapy, play or music therapy, and mutual storytelling.

Medications

Various medications are used to manage behavioral disorders in children and adolescents. Parents should understand that pharmacological management is most effective when accompanied by techniques to modify behavior.

Medications include central nervous system (CNS) stimulants, selective reuptake inhibitors (SNRIs), tricyclic antidepressants (TCAs), alpha$_2$–adrenergic agonists, atypical antipsychotics, and selective serotonin reuptake inhibitors (SSRIs).

Other medications used to treat the manifestations of intermittent explosive disorder include lithium, mood-stabilizing antiepileptics, and beta-adrenergic blockers.

CNS stimulants

SELECT PROTOTYPE MEDICATION: Methylphenidate

OTHER MEDICATIONS
- Amphetamine mixture
- Dextroamphetamine
- Dexmethylphenidate
- Lisdexamfetamine dimesylate

PURPOSE Q_EBP

EXPECTED PHARMACOLOGICAL ACTION: These medications raise the levels of norepinephrine and dopamine into the central nervous system.

THERAPEUTIC USES: ADHD in children and adults

COMPLICATIONS

CNS stimulation (insomnia, restlessness)

NURSING ACTIONS
- Decrease dosage as prescribed.
- Administer the last dose of the day before 4 p.m.

CLIENT EDUCATION
- Observe for effects and notify the provider if they occur.
- Decrease use of items that contain caffeine (coffee, tea, cola, chocolate).

Weight loss related to reduced appetite; growth suppression

NURSING ACTIONS
- Monitor the client's height and weight and compare with baseline height and weight.
- Consult with the provider regarding giving the client a "holiday" from the medication.
- Administer medication during or after meals.

CLIENT EDUCATION: Eat at regular meal times and avoid unhealthy food choices.

Cardiovascular effects

- Dysrhythmias, chest pain, high blood pressure
- Can increase the risk of sudden death in clients who have heart abnormalities

NURSING ACTIONS
- Monitor vital signs and ECG.
- Advise the client to observe for effects and to notify the provider if they occur.

Development of psychotic manifestations, (hallucinations and paranoia)

CLIENT EDUCATION: Report manifestations immediately and discontinue the medication.

Withdrawal reaction

Headache, nausea, vomiting, muscle weakness, and depression.

CLIENT EDUCATION: Avoid abrupt cessation of the medication.

Hypersensitivity skin reaction to transdermal methylphenidate: hives, papules

CLIENT EDUCATION: Remove the patch and notify the provider.

Toxicity

Dizziness, palpitations, hypertension, hallucinations, seizures

NURSING ACTIONS
- Treat hallucinations with chlorpromazine.
- Treat seizures with diazepam.
- Administer fluids.

CONTRAINDICATIONS/PRECAUTIONS

- Contraindicated in clients who have a history of substance use disorder, cardiovascular disorders, severe anxiety, and psychosis
- CNS stimulants are teratogenic medications.

INTERACTIONS

MAOIs

Concurrent use can cause hypertensive crisis.

NURSING ACTIONS: Discontinue MAOIs and wait at least 14 days prior to administering amphetamine medications.

Caffeine

Concurrent use can cause an increase in CNS stimulant effects.

NURSING ACTIONS: Instruct the client to avoid foods and beverages that contain caffeine.

Phenytoin, warfarin and phenobarbital

Methylphenidate inhibits metabolism of these medications, leading to increased blood levels.

NURSING ACTIONS
- Monitor for adverse effects (CNS depression, bleeding).
- Caution with concurrent use of these medications

OTC cold and decongestant medications

Concurrent use can lead to increased CNS stimulation.

CLIENT EDUCATION: Avoid the use of these OTC medications.

NURSING ADMINISTRATION Qpcc

- Advise clients to swallow sustained-release tablets whole and to not chew or crush them.
- Teach the client the importance of administering the medication on a regular schedule. Medications are available in regular or extended-release formulas.
- Oral tablets should be given 30 to 45 min before meals, with the last dose of the day given by 4 p.m. Administer oral suspension regardless of meals, and shake the container for 10 seconds before measuring the dose.
- Teach clients who use transdermal medication to place the patch on one hip daily in the morning, and leave it in place no longer than 9 hr. Alternate hips daily. Flush the patch down the toilet after removal.
- Advise parents that full response to medications can take up to 6 weeks.
- Teach client to avoid use of all OTC medications unless approved by the provider.
- Advise client to avoid alcohol use while taking this medication.
- Instruct parents and clients that ADHD is not cured by the medication. Management in conjunction with an overall treatment plan that includes family and cognitive therapy will improve outcomes. QEBP
- Instruct parents that these medications have special handling procedures controlled by federal law. Handwritten prescriptions are required for medication refills.
- Instruct parents regarding safety and storage of medications.
- Advise parents that use of these medications causes a high potential for development of a substance use disorder, especially in adolescents.

NURSING EVALUATION OF MEDICATION EFFECTIVENESS

Depending on therapeutic intent, effectiveness can be evidenced by improvement of manifestations of ADHD (an increased ability to focus and complete tasks, interact with peers, and manage impulsivity).

Selective norepinephrine reuptake inhibitors

SELECT PROTOTYPE MEDICATION: Atomoxetine

OTHER MEDICATION: Bupropion

PURPOSE QEBP

EXPECTED PHARMACOLOGICAL ACTION: Block reuptake of norepinephrine at synapses in the CNS. Atomoxetine is not a stimulant medication.

THERAPEUTIC USES: ADHD in children and adults

COMPLICATIONS Qs

Usually tolerated well with minimal adverse effects

Appetite/growth suppression, weight loss

NURSING ACTIONS
- Monitor height and weight and compare with baseline.
- Administer medication with or after meals.
- Encourage children to eat at regular meal times and avoid unhealthy food choices.

GI effects (nausea, vomiting, upper abdominal pain)

CLIENT EDUCATION: Take the medication with food if GI effects occur.

Suicidal ideation (in children and adolescents)

NURSING ACTIONS: Monitor the client for indications of depression.

CLIENT EDUCATION: Report changes in mood, excessive sleeping, agitation, and irritability.

Hepatotoxicity

CLIENT EDUCATION: Report indications of liver damage (flu-like manifestations, yellowing skin, abdominal pain).

CNS effects (headache, insomnia, irritability)

NURSING ACTIONS
- Decrease dosage as prescribed.
- Administer the last dose of the day before 4 p.m.

CLIENT EDUCATION
- Observe for effects, and notify the provider if they occur.
- Decrease use of items that contain caffeine (coffee, tea, cola, chocolate).

CONTRAINDICATIONS/PRECAUTIONS

- Use cautiously in clients who have cardiovascular disorders. Qs
- Contraindicated in clients who have suicidal ideation
- Atomoxetine is contraindicated for clients who have angle-closure glaucoma or pheochromocytoma.

INTERACTIONS

MAOIs

Concurrent use can cause hypertensive crisis.

CLIENT EDUCATION: Discontinue MAOIs and wait at least 14 days prior to administering amphetamine medications.

Paroxetine, fluoxetine, or quinidine gluconate

These medications inhibit metabolizing enzymes, thereby increasing levels of atomoxetine.

NURSING ACTIONS: Concurrent use can require a reduction in the dosage of atomoxetine.

CLIENT EDUCATION: Watch for and report increased adverse effects of atomoxetine.

NURSING ADMINISTRATION

- Note any changes in the client related to dosing and timing of medications.
- Administer the medication in one daily dose in the morning or in two divided doses, morning and afternoon, with or without food.

CLIENT EDUCATION

- Initial response takes a few days to develop, but maximal therapeutic effects can take up to 6 weeks to fully develop.
- Avoid alcohol use while taking this medication.
- Avoid use of all OTC medications unless approved by provider.

NURSING EVALUATION OF MEDICATION EFFECTIVENESS

Depending on therapeutic intent, effectiveness can be evidenced by improvement of the manifestations of ADHD (increase in ability to focus and complete tasks, interact with peers, and manage impulsivity).

Tricyclic antidepressants

SELECT PROTOTYPE MEDICATION: Desipramine

OTHER MEDICATIONS
- Imipramine
- Clomipramine

PURPOSE

EXPECTED PHARMACOLOGICAL ACTION: These medications block reuptake of norepinephrine and serotonin in the synaptic space, thereby intensifying the effects of these neurotransmitters.

THERAPEUTIC USES IN CHILDREN
- Depression
- Autism spectrum disorder
- ADHD
- Panic disorder, separation anxiety disorder
- Social phobia
- OCD

COMPLICATIONS Qs

Orthostatic hypotension

NURSING ACTIONS
- Monitor blood pressure with first dose.
- If orthostatic hypotension occurs, instruct the client to change positions slowly.

Anticholinergic effects

- Dry mouth
- Blurred vision
- Photophobia
- Urinary hesitancy or retention
- Constipation
- Tachycardia

CLIENT EDUCATION
- Methods to minimize anticholinergic effects include:
  - Chewing sugarless gum
  - Sipping water
  - Wearing sunglasses when outdoors
  - Eating foods high in fiber
  - Increasing fluid intake to at least 2 to 3 L/day from beverages and other food sources
  - Voiding just before taking the medication
- Notify the provider if effects become intolerable.

Weight gain related to increased appetite

NURSING ACTIONS: Monitor client weight.

Sedation

CLIENT EDUCATION
- Sedative effects should diminish over time.
- Avoid hazardous activities (driving) if sedation is excessive.
- Take the medication at bedtime to minimize daytime sleepiness and to promote sleep. Taking the medication at bedtime minimizes adverse effects during the day.

Toxicity

Resulting in cholinergic blockade and cardiac toxicity evidenced by dysrhythmias, mental confusion, and agitation, followed by seizures, coma, and possible death

NURSING ACTIONS
- Give a client who is acutely ill a 1-week supply of medication.
- Obtain baseline ECG.
- Monitor vital signs frequently.
- Monitor for toxicity.
- Notify the provider if indications of toxicity occur.

Decreased seizure threshold

NURSING ACTIONS: Monitor clients who have seizure disorders.

Excessive sweating

CLIENT EDUCATION: Monitor for this adverse effect, and perform frequent linen changes.

CONTRAINDICATIONS/PRECAUTIONS

- Desipramine, clomipramine, and imipramine teratogenic medications Qs
- This medication is contraindicated for clients who have had a recent MI or a history of heart failure or prolonged QT complex.
- Use this medication cautiously in clients who have seizure disorders, coronary artery disease; diabetes; liver, kidney, and respiratory disorders; urinary retention and obstruction; angle closure glaucoma; benign prostatic hypertrophy; and hyperthyroidism.
- TCAs can increase suicide risk and can be lethal if excessive dosages are taken.

INTERACTIONS

MAOIs

Concurrent use can cause severe hypertension.

NURSING ACTIONS: Do not administer concurrently with MAOIs. Wait 14 days after discontinuing MAOIs to start these medications.

Antihistamines and other anticholinergic agents

Concurrent use can cause additive anticholinergic effects.

NURSING ACTIONS: Do not administer concurrently with antihistamines.

Epinephrine and dopamine (direct-acting sympathomimetics)

Concurrent use can cause hypertensive effect.

NURSING ACTIONS: Do not administer these medications concurrently with TCAs.

Alcohol, benzodiazepines, opioids, and antihistamines

Concurrent use can cause additive CNS depression.

CLIENT EDUCATION: Avoid other CNS depressants while taking a TCA.

NURSING ADMINISTRATION Qpcc

- Instruct the client's parents to administer this medication as prescribed on a daily basis to establish therapeutic plasma levels.
- Assist with medication regimen adherence by informing the client and parents that it can take 1 to 3 weeks to experience initial therapeutic effects. Full therapeutic effects can take around 6 weeks.
- Instruct the client and parents on the importance of continuing therapy after improvement in manifestations. Sudden discontinuation of the medication can result in relapse.
- Take medication at bedtime to prevent daytime drowsiness.
- Due to high suicide potential, give only a 1-week supply of medication for a client who is acutely ill, and then only give a 1-month supply of medication at a time. Qs

NURSING EVALUATION OF MEDICATION EFFECTIVENESS

Depending on therapeutic intent, effectiveness can be evidenced by the following.

FOR CLIENTS WHO HAVE DEPRESSION
- Verbalization of improvement in mood
- Improved sleeping and eating habits
- Increased interaction with peers

FOR CLIENTS WHO HAVE AUTISM SPECTRUM DISORDER
- Decreased anger
- Decreased compulsive behavior

FOR CLIENTS WHO HAVE ADHD
- Decreased hyperactivity
- Greater ability to pay attention

FOR CLIENTS WHO HAVE OCD, PANIC, AND ANXIETY DISORDERS
- Reduced levels of anxiety
- Increased ability to recognize manifestations and triggers of disorder
- Ability to manage episodes of disorder
- Ability to perform self-care
- Increased interaction with peers
- Ability to assume usual role

Alpha₂-adrenergic agonists

SELECT PROTOTYPE MEDICATION: Guanfacine

OTHER MEDICATION: Clonidine

PURPOSE Q EBP

EXPECTED PHARMACOLOGICAL ACTION: The action of alpha2-adrenergic agonists is not completely understood; however, they are known to activate presynaptic alpha₂-adrenergic receptors within the brain.

THERAPEUTIC USES

- ADHD
- Tic disorders
- Conduct and oppositional defiant disorders

COMPLICATIONS

CNS effects (sedation, drowsiness, fatigue)

NURSING ACTIONS: Monitor for these adverse effects and report their occurrence to the provider.

CLIENT EDUCATION: Avoid hazardous activities.

Cardiovascular effects (hypotension, bradycardia)

NURSING ACTIONS: Monitor blood pressure and pulse, especially during initial treatment.

CLIENT EDUCATION: Abrupt discontinuation of medication can cause rebound hypertension.

Weight gain

NURSING ACTIONS
- Monitor client's weight.
- Encourage clients to participate in regular exercise and to follow a healthy, well-balanced diet.

GI effects

Nausea, vomiting, constipation, dry mouth

NURSING ACTIONS
- Monitor for these adverse effects and report their occurrence to the provider.
- Suggest that the client use the following strategies to prevent or minimize GI effects.
  - Chewing sugarless gum
  - Sipping water
  - Eating foods high in fiber
  - Participating in regular exercise
  - Increasing fluid intake to at least 2 to 3 L/day from beverages and other food sources

CONTRAINDICATIONS/PRECAUTIONS

- Safety has not been established for use of guanfacine or clonidine in children younger than 6 years old.
- Use cautiously in clients who have cardiac disease. Q s

INTERACTIONS

CNS depressants, including alcohol, can increase CNS effects.
NURSING ACTIONS: Avoid concurrent use.

Antihypertensives can worsen hypotension.
NURSING ACTIONS: Avoid concurrent use.

Foods with high-fat content increase guanfacine absorption.
NURSING ACTIONS: Avoid taking medication with a high-fat meal.

NURSING ADMINISTRATION

- Assess use of alcohol and CNS depressants, especially with adolescent clients. Q s
- Monitor blood pressure and pulse at baseline, with initial treatment and with each dosage change.

CLIENT EDUCATION
- Avoid abrupt discontinuation of medication, which can result in rebound hypertension. Medication should be tapered according to a prescribed dosage schedule when discontinuing treatment.
- Do not chew, crush, or split extended-release preparations.

NURSING EVALUATION OF MEDICATION EFFECTIVENESS

Depending on therapeutic intent, effectiveness can be evidenced by improvement of manifestations of ADHD (increase in ability to focus and complete tasks, interact with peers, and manage impulsivity).

Atypical antipsychotics

SELECT PROTOTYPE MEDICATION: Risperidone

OTHER MEDICATION
- Olanzapine
- Aripiprazole
- Quetiapine

PURPOSE Q EBP

EXPECTED PHARMACOLOGICAL ACTION: These antipsychotic agents work mainly by blocking serotonin and, to a lesser degree, dopamine receptors. These medications also block receptors for norepinephrine, histamine, and acetylcholine.

THERAPEUTIC USES
- Autism spectrum disorder
- Conduct disorder
- OCD
- Relief of psychotic manifestations

COMPLICATIONS

Diabetes mellitus

New onset of diabetes or loss of glucose control in clients who have diabetes

NURSING ACTIONS
- Obtain baseline fasting blood glucose, and monitor periodically throughout treatment.
- Instruct the client to report indications (increased thirst, urination, and appetite).

Weight gain

CLIENT EDUCATION: Follow a healthy, low-calorie diet; engage in regular exercise; and monitor weight gain.

Hypercholesterolemia

With increased risk for hypertension and other cardiovascular disease

NURSING ACTIONS: Monitor cholesterol, triglycerides, and blood glucose if weight gain is more than 14 kg (30 lb).

Orthostatic hypotension

NURSING ACTIONS: Monitor blood pressure with first dose, and instruct the client to change positions slowly if orthostatic hypotension occurs.

Anticholinergic effects

Urinary retention or hesitancy, dry mouth

NURSING ACTIONS: Monitor for these adverse effects, and report their occurrence to the provider.

CLIENT EDUCATION: Use measures to relieve dry mouth (sipping fluids throughout the day).

Agitation, dizziness, sedation, and sleep disruption

NURSING ACTIONS
- Monitor for these adverse effects and report their occurrence to the provider.
- Administer an alternative medication if prescribed.

Mild extrapyramidal adverse effects (tremor)

NURSING ACTIONS: Monitor for and teach clients to recognize EPS. These effects are usually dose-related.

CONTRAINDICATIONS/PRECAUTIONS

- Be aware of possible alcohol use in the adolescent client. Instruct clients to avoid the use of alcohol. Qs
- Use cautiously in clients who have cardiovascular disease, seizures, or diabetes. Clients who have diabetes should have a baseline fasting blood sugar, and blood glucose should be monitored carefully.

INTERACTIONS

CNS depressants
- Additive CNS depression occurs with concurrent use of alcohol, opioids, antihistamines.
- CLIENT EDUCATION
  - Avoid alcohol and other medications that cause CNS depression.
  - Avoid hazardous activities (driving).

Levodopa
- By activating dopamine receptors, levodopa counteracts the effects of antipsychotic agents.
- NURSING ACTIONS: Avoid concurrent use of levodopa and other direct dopamine receptor agonists.

TCAs, amiodarone, and clarithromycin prolong QT interval, thereby increasing the risk of cardiac dysrhythmias.
NURSING ACTIONS: Avoid concurrent use of these medications.

Barbiturates and phenytoin promote hepatic drug-metabolizing enzymes, thereby decreasing drug levels of quetiapine.
NURSING ACTIONS: Monitor medication for effectiveness.

Fluconazole and other medications that inhibit CYP3A4 inhibit hepatic drug-metabolizing enzymes, thereby increasing drug levels of aripiprazole, and quetiapine.
NURSING ACTIONS: Monitor for adverse medication effects.

NURSING ADMINISTRATION Qpcc

- Administer by oral or IM route.
  - Risperidone is available in an oral solution and quick-dissolving tablets for ease in administration.
  - Olanzapine is available in an orally disintegrating tablet for ease in administration.
  - Quetiapine is available for use in adolescents as an immediate-release tablet.
  - Aripiprazole is available for adolescents as a tablet to swallow, an orally-disintegrating table, or oral solution.
- Medications may be taken without regard to food.

CLIENT EDUCATION: Low doses of medication are given initially and are then gradually increased.

NURSING EVALUATION OF MEDICATION EFFECTIVENESS

Depending on therapeutic intent, effectiveness can be evidenced by the following.

FOR CLIENTS WHO HAVE AUTISM SPECTRUM DISORDER
- Reduction of hyperactivity
- Improvement in mood

FOR CLIENTS WHO HAVE CONDUCT DISORDER: Decreased aggressiveness

FOR CLIENTS WHO HAVE OCD
- Reduced levels of anxiety
- Ability to manage compulsive actions
- Ability to perform self-care
- Increased interaction with peers
- Ability to assume usual role

FOR CLIENTS WHO HAVE ADHD
Reduction in hyperactivity and impulsivity

Selective serotonin reuptake inhibitors

SELECT PROTOTYPE MEDICATION
- Fluoxetine
- Sertraline
- Fluvoxamine

PURPOSE QEBP

EXPECTED PHARMACOLOGICAL ACTION: SSRIs work by blocking the synaptic reuptake of serotonin, allowing more serotonin to stay at the junction of the neurons.

THERAPEUTIC USES
- Intermittent explosive disorder
- Autism spectrum disorder
- Obsessive-compulsive disorder
- Major depressive disorder
- Bulimia nervosa
- Generalized anxiety disorder

COMPLICATIONS

Agitation, anxiety, sleep disturbance, tremors, and tension headache

NURSING ACTIONS: Monitor for these adverse effects and report their occurrence to the provider. Agitation and hallucinations can indicate serotonin syndrome.

Weight changes

CLIENT EDUCATION
- Weigh weekly and report any significant weight change to the provider.
- Follow a healthy diet.

GI effects

Nausea, constipation or diarrhea, dry mouth

NURSING ACTIONS: Monitor for these adverse effects and report their occurrence to the provider.

CLIENT EDUCATION: Use measures to relieve dry mouth (sipping fluids throughout the day, chewing sugarless gum). Take with food to minimize GI distress.

CONTRAINDICATIONS/PRECAUTIONS

- SSRIs might increase suicidal ideation in children and adolescents. Qs
- Abrupt withdrawal of medication can lead to discontinuation syndrome (dizziness, insomnia, nervousness, irritability, agitation). Dose should be tapered.

INTERACTIONS

Concurrent use of MAOIs, SNRIs, buspirone, or St. John's wort can cause serotonin syndrome.
- CLIENT EDUCATION
  - Avoid concurrent use
  - Allow 2 weeks between fluoxetine and MAOI use.

NURSING ADMINISTRATION

- Sustained-release tablets should be taken whole and not chewed or crushed.
- Assist the client with medication regimen adherence by informing the client that the initial response occurs in 1 to 3 weeks, with maximum therapeutic effectiveness by 12 weeks.

CLIENT EDUCATION
- SSRIs may be taken with or without food. Sleep disturbances are minimized by taking the medication in the morning. QEBP
- Take the medication on a daily basis to establish therapeutic plasma levels.
- Do not abruptly stop taking the medication to avoid withdrawal syndrome.
- Report suicidal ideations to the provider.

NURSING EVALUATION OF MEDICATION EFFECTIVENESS

Depending on therapeutic intent, effectiveness can be evidenced by the following.

FOR CLIENTS WHO HAVE INTERMITTENT EXPLOSIVE DISORDER
- Reduction of hyperactivity
- Improvement in mood

FOR CLIENTS WHO HAVE CONDUCT DISORDER
Decreased aggressiveness

1. A nurse is collecting data during the admission of an adolescent client who has depression. Which of the following findings should the nurse expect? (Select all that apply.)

   A. Fear of being alone

   B. Substance use

   C. Weight gain

   D. Irritability

   E. Aggressiveness

2. A nurse is reinforcing teaching with a group of guardians about manifestations of conduct disorder. Which of the following findings should the nurse include? (Select all that apply.)

   A. Bullying of others

   B. Threats of suicide

   C. Law-breaking activities

   D. Narcissistic behavior

   E. Flat affect

3. Match the following manifestations with the appropriate mental health disorder for children or adolescents.

A. Attention deficit hyperactivity disorder	1. Recurrent temper outbursts that are severe and do not correlate with situation
B. Conduct disorder	2. Feeling of sadness
C. Depressive disorder	3. Limit testing
D. Disruptive mood dysregulation disorder	4. Demonstrates lack of remorse
E. Oppositional defiant disorder	5. Inability of a person to control behaviors requiring sustained attention

4. A nurse is reinforcing teaching with the adoptive parent of a preschool-age child who has a new diagnosis of ADHD. Which of the following statements should the nurse make?

   A. "Behaviors associated with ADHD are present prior to age 3."

   B. "This disorder is characterized by argumentativeness."

   C. "Below-average intellectual functioning is associated with ADHD."

   D. "Because of this disorder, your child is at an increased risk for injury."

5. A nurse is collecting data from a 4-year-old child for indications of autism spectrum disorder. Which of the following findings should the nurse expect?

   A. Impulsive behavior

   B. Repetitive counting

   C. Destructiveness

   D. Somatic problems

6. A nurse is assisting the guardians of a school-age child who has oppositional defiant disorder in identifying strategies to promote positive behavior. Which of the following strategies should the nurse recommend? (Select all that apply.)

   A. Allow the child to choose which behaviors are unacceptable.

   B. Use role-playing to act out unacceptable behavior.

   C. Develop a reward system for acceptable behavior.

   D. Encourage the child to participate in school sports.

   E. Be consistent when addressing unacceptable behavior.

7. A nurse is caring for a school-age child who has conduct disorder and a new prescription for methylphenidate transdermal patches. Which of the following information should the nurse provide about the medication?

   A. Apply the patch once daily at bedtime.

   B. Place the patch carefully in a trash can after removal.

   C. Apply the transdermal patch to the anterior waist area.

   D. Remove the patch each day after 9 hr.

8. A nurse is reinforcing education with an adolescent client who is to begin taking atomoxetine for ADHD. The nurse should instruct the client to monitor for which of the following adverse effects? (Select all that apply.)

   A. Somnolence

   B. Yellowing skin

   C. Increased appetite

   D. Fever

   E. Malaise

1. **B, D, E. CORRECT:** Substance use is an expected finding associated with depression. Irritability is an expected finding associated with depression. Aggressiveness is an expected finding associated with depression. Solitary play or work, rather than the fear of being alone, is an expected finding associated with depression. Loss of appetite and weight loss, not weight gain, are expected findings associated with depression.

   Ⓝ *NCLEX® Connection: Psychosocial Integrity, Mental Health Concepts*

2. **A, B, C. CORRECT:** Bullying behavior is an expected finding of conduct disorder. Suicidal ideation is an expected finding of conduct disorder. Law- and/or rule-breaking behavior is an expected finding of conduct disorder. Low self-esteem, rather than narcissism, is an expected finding of conduct disorder. Irritability and temper outbursts, rather than a flat affect, are expected findings of conduct disorder.

   Ⓝ *NCLEX® Connection: Psychosocial Integrity, Mental Health Concepts*

3. **A, 5; B, 4; C, 2; D, 1; E, 3**

   The nurse should recognize a manifestation of disruptive mood dysregulation disorder is recurrent temper outbursts that are severe and do not correlate with situations. Feelings of sadness are a finding associated with depressive disorder. Limit testing is associated with oppositional defiant disorder. A lack of remorse is a finding seen in conduct disorders. Inability of a person to control behaviors requiring sustained attention is associated with attention deficit hyperactivity disorder.

   Ⓝ *NCLEX® Connection: Psychosocial Integrity, Mental Health Concepts*

4. **D. CORRECT:** Inattentive or impulsive behavior increases the risk for injury in a child who has ADHD. Behaviors associated with ADHD are present before the age of 12. Argumentativeness is associated with oppositional defiant disorder rather than ADHD. Below-average intellectual functioning is associated with intellectual developmental disorder rather than ADHD.

   Ⓝ *NCLEX® Connection: Psychosocial Integrity, Mental Health Concepts*

5. **B. CORRECT:** Repetitive actions and strict routines are an indication of autism spectrum disorder. Impulsive behavior is an indication of ADHD rather than autism spectrum disorder. Destructiveness is an indication of conduct disorder rather than autism spectrum disorder. Somatic problems are an indication of posttraumatic stress disorder rather than autism spectrum disorder.

   Ⓝ *NCLEX® Connection: Psychosocial Integrity, Mental Health Concepts*

6. **C, D, E. CORRECT:** The guardians should have a method to reward the child for acceptable behavior, set clear limits on unacceptable behavior, be consistent, and encourage physical activity through which the child can use energy and obtain success.

   Ⓝ *NCLEX® Connection: Psychosocial Integrity, Behavioral Management*

7. **D. CORRECT:** The transdermal patch is applied once daily in the morning and is removed after 9 hr. For safety when discarding the transdermal preparation, the client should fold the patch and flush it down the toilet to prevent others from using it. The transdermal patch should be applied to a clean, dry area on the hip, and the waist area should be avoided.

   Ⓝ *NCLEX® Connection: Pharmacological Therapies, Medication Administration*

8. **B, D, E. CORRECT:** Yellowing skin is a potential indication of hepatotoxicity that the client should report to the provider. Fever and malaise is a potential indication of hepatotoxicity that the client should report to the provider. Insomnia, rather than somnolence, is an adverse effect that the client should report to the provider. Decreased appetite with resulting weight loss, rather than increased appetite, is a potential adverse effect that the client should report to the provider.

   Ⓝ *NCLEX® Connection: Pharmacological Therapies, Adverse Effects/Contraindications/Side Effects/Interactions*

Active Learning Scenario

A nurse is assisting with a peer group discussion with a group of high school students about primary prevention. Use the ATI Active Learning Template: Basic Concept to complete this item.

UNDERLYING PRINCIPLES: Identify the purpose of primary prevention.

NURSING INTERVENTIONS: Identify at least four primary prevention interventions.

Active Learning Scenario Key

Using the ATI Active Learning Template: Basic Concept

UNDERLYING PRINCIPLES: The purpose of primary prevention is to help the adolescent avoid risky behavior and to promote healthy behavior and effective coping.

NURSING INTERVENTIONS
- Assist clients in adopting a realistic view of their bodies.
- Promote positive self-esteem.
- Identify and reinforce the use of positive coping skills.
- Reinforce teaching about the use of gun and weapon control strategies.
- Emphasize the use of seat belts when in motor vehicles.
- Encourage the use of protective gear for high-impact sports.
- Reinforce teaching on contraceptives and the prevention of sexually transmitted infections.

Ⓝ *NCLEX® Connection: Health Promotion and Maintenance, Health Promotion/Disease Prevention*

NCLEX® Connections

When reviewing the following chapters, keep in mind the relevant topics and tasks of the NCLEX outline.

Psychosocial Integrity

ABUSE OR NEGLECT
Recognize risk factors for domestic, child or elder abuse or neglect and sexual abuse.

Provide a safe environment for an abused/neglected client.

Reinforce client teaching on coping strategies to prevent abuse or neglect.

Identify signs and symptoms of physical, psychological, or financial abuse in client.

CRISIS INTERVENTION
Identify client in crisis.

Identify client risk for self-injury and/or violence.

Assist in managing the care of angry and/or agitated client.

Use crisis intervention techniques to assist client in coping.

THERAPEUTIC COMMUNICATION: Use therapeutic communication techniques with client.

CHAPTER 23 *Suicide*

Suicide is the intentional act of killing oneself. A client who is suicidal can be ambivalent about death; interventions can make a difference. A client contemplating suicide believes that the act is the end to problems. Little concern is given to the aftermath or the ramifications to those left behind. Long-term therapy is needed for the survivors.

Suicidal ideation occurs when a client is having thoughts about committing suicide. Clients can have feelings of hopelessness, helplessness, and inner pain.

MYTHS REGARDING SUICIDE

- People who talk about suicide never commit it.
- People who are suicidal only want to hurt themselves, not others.
- There is no way to help someone who really wants to kill themselves.
- Asking a client about suicide will cause the suicidal individual to actually commit suicide.
- Ignoring verbal threats of killing oneself, or challenging a person to carry out plans to kill oneself, will reduce the individual's use of these behaviors.
- People who talk about suicide are only trying to get attention.

DATA COLLECTION

RISK FACTORS

While females are more likely to attempt suicide, adolescent, middle, and older adult males are more likely to have died by suicide. Other individuals at increased risk for suicide include active military personnel/veterans; those who are lesbian, gay, bisexual, or transgender; and people who have a comorbid mental illness (depressive disorders, substance use disorders, schizophrenia, bipolar disorder, and personality disorders).

OLDER ADULT CLIENTS Ⓖ

- Untreated depression
- Loss of employment and finances
- Feelings of isolation, powerlessness
- Prior attempts at suicide (Older adult clients are more likely to succeed.)
- Change in functional ability
- Declining physical health
- Alcohol or other substance use disorder
- Loss of loved ones

BIOLOGICAL FACTORS

- Family history of suicide
- Physical disorders (AIDS, cancer, cardiovascular disease, stroke, chronic kidney disease, cirrhosis, dementia, epilepsy, head injury, Huntington's disease, and multiple sclerosis)

PSYCHOSOCIAL FACTORS

- Sense of hopelessness
- Intense emotions (rage, anger, or guilt)
- Poor interpersonal relationships at home, school, and work
- Developmental stressors, such as those experienced by adolescents
- History of trauma/abuse

CULTURAL FACTORS: Whites are at the highest risk than any other culture and have the highest incidence of completed suicides. This is followed by Native Americans, African Americans, Asian Americans, and Hispanic Americans.

ENVIRONMENTAL FACTORS

- Access to lethal methods, such as firearms
- Lack of access to adequate mental health care
- Unemployment

PROTECTIVE FACTORS

- Feelings of responsibility toward partner and children
- Current pregnancy
- Religious and cultural beliefs
- Overall satisfaction with life
- Presence of adequate social support
- Effective coping and problem-solving skills
- Access to adequate medical care

EXPECTED FINDINGS

- Monitor carefully for verbal and nonverbal clues. It is essential to ask the client if they are thinking of suicide. This will not give the client the idea to commit suicide. Qs
- Suicidal comments usually are made to someone that the client perceives as supportive.
- Monitor for potential suicide risk using the Suicide Assessment Five-step Evaluation and Triage (SAFE-T). Qebp
- Comments or signals can be overt (direct) or covert (indirect).
  - **Overt comment:** "There is just no reason for me to go on living."
  - **Covert comment:** "Everything is looking pretty grim for me."
- Monitor the client's suicide plan. Qs
  - Does the client have a plan?
  - How lethal is the plan?
  - Can the client describe the plan exactly?
  - Does the client have access to the intended method?
  - Has the client's mood changed? A sudden change in mood from sad and depressed to happy and peaceful can indicate a client's intention to commit suicide.

PHYSICAL FINDINGS: Lacerations, scratches, and scars that could indicate previous attempts at self-harm

SERIOUS WARNING SIGNS

- Having sudden and extreme mood swings
- Developing a suicide plan, such as collecting pills, buying a gun, etc.
- Complaining about feeling great guilt or shame
- Increasing use of drugs or alcohol
- Behaving anxious or agitated
- Changing eating or sleeping habits
- Displaying rage or talking about seeking revenge

PATIENT-CENTERED CARE

NURSING CARE

Nursing care consists of primary, secondary, and tertiary interventions.

- **Primary interventions** focus on suicide prevention through the use of community education and screenings to identify individuals at risk.
- **Secondary interventions** focus on suicide prevention for an individual client who is having an acute suicidal crisis. Suicide precautions are included in this level of intervention.
- **Tertiary interventions** focus on providing support and assistance to survivors of a client who died by suicide.

Suicide precautions

Suicide precautions include milieu therapy within the facility.

- Initiate one-on-one constant supervision around the clock, always having the client in sight and close. Documentation should indicate which staff member is accountable for the client, with specific start and stop times. There is an increased risk for suicide during staff rotation times.
- Document the client's location, mood, quoted statements, and behavior every 15 min or per facility protocol.
- Search the client's belongings with the client present. Remove all glass, metal silverware, electrical cords, vases, belts, shoelaces, metal nail files, tweezers, matches, razors, perfume, shampoo, plastic bags, and other potentially harmful items from the client's room and vicinity.
- Allow the client to use only plastic eating utensils. Count utensils when brought into and out of the client's room.
- Check the environment for possible hazards (windows that open, overhead pipes that are easily accessible, non-breakaway shower rods, non-recessed shower nozzles).
- Ensure that the client's hands are always visible, even when sleeping.

- Do not assign to a private room and keep door open at all times.
- Ensure that the client swallows all medications. Clients can try to hoard medication until there is enough for a suicide attempt.
- Identify whether the client's current medications can be lethal with exceeding the prescribed dose. If so, collaborate with the provider to have less dangerous medications substituted if possible.
- Restrict visitors from bringing possibly harmful items to the client.
- Collaborate with client to develop a safety plan.

Self-assessment

- The nurse must determine how they feel personally about suicide.
- The nurse must become comfortable asking personal questions about suicidal ideation and following up on client's answers.
- Death of a client by suicide can cause health care professionals to experience hopelessness, helplessness, ambivalence, anger, anxiety, avoidance, and denial.
- Nurses who work with clients who have suicidal ideation can benefit personally by debriefing, sharing, and collaborating with other health professionals.

MEDICATIONS

Classifications of medications to prevent suicide include the following.

Antidepressants: Selective serotonin reuptake inhibitors

- Citalopram
- Fluoxetine
- Sertraline

NURSING ACTIONS

- Decreased risk of lethal toxicity compared with other categories of antidepressants
- Do not stop taking medication suddenly.
- Medications can take 1 to 3 weeks for therapeutic effects for initial response with up to 2 months for maximal response.
- Avoid hazardous activities (driving, operating heavy equipment/machinery) until medication adverse effects are known. Adverse effects can include nausea, headache, and central nervous system (CNS) stimulation (agitation, insomnia, anxiety).
- Sexual dysfunction can occur. Notify the provider if effects are intolerable.
- Follow a healthy diet, as weight gain can occur with long-term use.
- Monitor for indications of increased depression and intent of suicide.

Sedative hypnotic anxiolytics (benzodiazepines)

- Diazepam
- Lorazepam

CLIENT EDUCATION
- Observe for CNS depression (sedation, lightheadedness, ataxia, and decreased cognitive function).
- Avoid the use of other CNS depressants (alcohol).
- Avoid hazardous activities (driving, operating heavy equipment/machinery).
- Caffeine interferes with the desired effects of the medication.
- If seeking to discontinue benzodiazepine, seek the advice of a provider. Do not abruptly discontinue these medications. The provider should gradually taper the dosage over several weeks.

Mood stabilizers

Lithium carbonate

NURSING ACTIONS
- Maintain a healthy diet, and exercise regularly to minimize weight gain.
- Maintain fluid intake of 2 to 3 L/day from food and beverage sources.
- Maintain adequate sodium intake.

CLIENT EDUCATION
- Minimize gastrointestinal effects by taking medication with food or milk.
- Comply with laboratory appointments needed to monitor lithium effectiveness and adverse effects.

Second-generation antipsychotics

- Risperidone
- Olanzapine
- Clozapine

NURSING ACTIONS: Preferred over first-generation antipsychotics due to decreased adverse effects.

CLIENT EDUCATION
- To minimize weight gain, maintain a healthy diet and exercise regularly.
- Report clinical findings of agitation, dizziness, sedation, and sleep disruption to the provider, as the medication might need to be changed.

THERAPEUTIC PROCEDURES

Therapeutic communication

- When questioning the client about suicide, always use a follow-up question if the first answer is negative. For example, the client says, "I'm feeling completely hopeless." The nurse says, "Are you thinking of suicide?" Client: "No, I'm just sad." Nurse: "I can see you're very sad. Are you thinking about hurting yourself?" Client: "Well, I've thought about it a lot." Qs
- Establish a trusting therapeutic relationship.
- Limit the amount of time an at-risk client spends alone.
- Involve significant others in the treatment plan.
- Carry out treatment plans for the client who has a comorbid disorder (a dual diagnosis of substance use disorder).

Electroconvulsive therapy (ECT)

ECT is effective in decreasing suicidal ideation in clients who have a depressive or psychotic disorder.

CLIENT EDUCATION

Assist the client to develop a support-system list with specific names, agencies, and telephone numbers that the client can call in case of an emergency.

CARE AFTER DISCHARGE
Agree to a no-suicide contract, which is a verbal or written agreement made to not harm themselves but instead to seek help. Qpcc
- A no-suicide contract is not legally binding and should only be used according to facility policy.
- A no-suicide contract can be beneficial, but it should not replace other suicide prevention strategies.
- A no-suicide contract can be used as a tool to develop and maintain trust between the nurse and the client.
- A no-suicide contract is discouraged for clients who are in crisis, under the influence of substances, psychotic, very impulsive, and/or very angry/agitated.

Active Learning Scenario

A nurse is caring for a client who has a new prescription for sertraline. Use the ATI Active Learning Template: Medication to complete this item.

COMPLICATIONS: Identify four adverse effects.

CLIENT EDUCATION: Describe at least three teaching points to reinforce.

Application Exercises

1. A nurse is collecting data from a client who has major depressive disorder. The nurse should identify which of the following client statements as an overt comment about suicide? (Select all that apply.)

   A. "My family will be better off if I'm dead."

   B. "The stress in my life is too much to handle."

   C. "I wish my life was over."

   D. "I don't feel like I can ever be happy again."

   E. "If I kill myself, then my problems will go away."

2. A nurse is caring for a client who states, "I plan to commit suicide." Which of the following findings should the nurse identify as the priority?

   A. Client's educational and economic background

   B. Lethality of the method and availability of means

   C. Quality of the client's social support

   D. Client's insight into the reasons for the decision

3. A nurse is assisting with the development of protocols to address the increasing number of suicide attempts in the community. Which of the following interventions should the nurse include as a primary intervention? (Select all that apply.)

   A. Conducting a suicide-risk screening on all new clients

   B. Creating a support group for family members of clients who died by suicide

   C. Informing high school teens about suicide prevention

   D. Initiating one-on-one observation for a client who has current suicidal ideation

   E. Reinforcing teaching middle-school educators about warning indicators of suicide

4. A nurse is caring for a client who is on suicide precautions. Which of the following interventions should the nurse contribute to the plan of care?

   A. Assign the client to a private room.

   B. Document the client's behavior every hour.

   C. Allow the client to keep perfume in their room.

   D. Ensure that the client swallows medication.

5. A nurse is assisting in conducting a class for a group of newly licensed nurses on caring for clients who are at risk for suicide. Which of the following information should the nurse include in the teaching?

   A. A client's verbal threat of suicide is attention-seeking behavior.

   B. Interventions are ineffective for clients who really want to commit suicide.

   C. Using the term *suicide* increases the client's risk for a suicide attempt.

   D. A no-suicide contract decreases the client's risk for suicide.

Application Exercises Key

1. **A, C, E. CORRECT:** An overt comment about suicide is when the client directly talks about their perception of an outcome of their death. A covert comment is when the client identifies a problem but does not directly talk about suicide. The nurse should assess the client further for a suicide plan.

   Ⓝ *NCLEX® Connection: Psychosocial Integrity, Crisis Intervention*

2. **B. CORRECT:** The greatest risk to the client is self-harm as a result of carrying out a suicide plan. The priority assessment is to determine how lethal the method is, how available the method is, and how detailed the plan is.

   Ⓝ *NCLEX® Connection: Psychosocial Integrity, Crisis Intervention*

3. **C, E. CORRECT:** Primary interventions include suicide prevention through the use of community education. Informing high school teens about suicide prevention is an example of a primary intervention. Reinforcing teaching with middle-school teachers to recognize the warning indicators of suicide is an example of a primary intervention. Initiating one-on-one observation for a client who has current suicidal ideation is an example of a secondary intervention. Creating a support group for family members of clients who died by suicide is an example of a tertiary intervention.

   Ⓝ *NCLEX® Connection: Psychosocial Integrity, Crisis Intervention*

4. **D. CORRECT:** When assisting with planning care, the nurse should ensure that the client swallows medication to prevent hoarding of medication for an attempt to exceed the prescribed dose. Clients who are suicidal should not be assigned a private room. Client's behavior should be documented every 15 min or according to facility policy. Remove perfume from the client's room.

   Ⓝ *NCLEX® Connection: Psychosocial Integrity, Crisis Intervention*

5. **D. CORRECT:** The use of a no-suicide contract decreases the client's risk for suicide by promoting and maintaining trust between the nurse and the client. However, it should not replace other suicide prevention strategies. It is a myth that a threat of suicide or suicide attempt is attention-seeking behavior. It is a myth that interventions are ineffective for clients who really want to commit suicide. Suicide precautions are shown to be effective in reducing the risk of a completed suicide. It is a myth that using the term suicide increases the client's risk for a suicide attempt. Discuss suicide openly with the client.

   Ⓝ *NCLEX® Connection: Health Promotion and Maintenance, High-Risk Behaviors*

Active Learning Scenario Key

Using the ATI Active Learning Template: Medication

ADVERSE EFFECTS
- Nausea
- Headache
- Central nervous system stimulation (agitation, insomnia, anxiety)
- Sexual dysfunction

CLIENT EDUCATION
- Do not stop taking medication suddenly.
- Medications can take 1 to 3 weeks for therapeutic effects for initial response with up to 2 months for maximal response.
- Avoid hazardous activities (driving, operating heavy equipment/machinery) until medication adverse effects are known.
- Follow a healthy diet, as weight gain can occur with long-term use.
- Monitor for indications of increased depression and intent of suicide.

Ⓝ *NCLEX® Connection: Pharmacological Therapies, Adverse Effects/Contraindications/Side Effects/Interactions*

UNIT 5   CRITICAL MENTAL HEALTH CONCERNS

CHAPTER 24 *Crisis and Anger Management*

A crisis is an acute, time-limited (usually lasting 4 to 6 weeks) event during which a client experiences an emotional response that cannot be managed with the client's normal coping mechanisms. During crisis intervention, it is assumed that the client was well-functioning and mentally healthy.

Everyone experiences crises. A crisis is not pathological but represents a struggle for equilibrium and adaptation. Crises are also personal in nature. What might be considered a crisis for one person might not be so for another. During crises, the individual will experience either psychological deterioration or growth.

COMMON CRISIS CHARACTERISTICS

- Experiencing a sudden event with little or no time to prepare
- Perception of the event as overwhelming or life-threatening
- Loss or decrease in communication with significant others
- Sense of displacement from the familiar
- An actual or perceived loss

TYPES OF CRISES

Situational/external: Often unanticipated loss or change experienced in everyday, often unanticipated, life events (divorce or job change)

Maturational/internal: Achieving new developmental stages, which requires learning additional coping mechanisms. Examples include getting married or retiring.

Adventitious
- The occurrence of natural disasters, crimes, or national disasters
- People in communities with large-scale psychological trauma caused by natural disasters

DATA COLLECTION

The nursing history should include the following.
- Presence of suicidal or homicidal ideation requiring possible admission to an acute facility Qs
- The client's perception of the precipitating event
- Cultural or religious needs of the client
- Support system
- Present coping skills
- Disorganization
- Feeling of being overwhelmed and anxiety
- Inadequate problem-solving
- Possible anger or aggression

RISK FACTORS

- Accumulation of unresolved losses
- Current life stressors
- Concurrent mental and physical health issues
- Excessive fatigue or pain
- Age and developmental stage

PROTECTIVE FACTORS

- Support system
- Prior experience with stress/crisis

EXPECTED FINDINGS

Phases of a crisis

Phase 1: Escalating anxiety from a threat activates increased defense responses.

Phase 2: Anxiety continues escalating as defense responses fail, functioning becomes disorganized, and the client resorts to trial-and-error attempts to resolve anxiety.

Phase 3: Trial-and-error methods of resolution fail, and the client's anxiety escalates to severe or panic levels, leading to flight or withdrawal behaviors.

Phase 4: The client experiences overwhelming anxiety that can lead to anguish and apprehension, feelings of powerlessness and being overwhelmed, dissociative findings (depersonalization, detachment from reality), depression, confusion, and/or violence against others or self.

PATIENT-CENTERED CARE

NURSING CARE

- Crisis intervention is designed to provide rapid assistance for individuals or groups who have an urgent need. Care is directed at the resolution of the immediate problem causing a crisis.
- The initial task of the nurse is to promote a sense of safety for the client and protect the client by monitoring the client's potential for suicide or homicide. Qs
  - Assist with admission to an inpatient facility, as needed for clients who have suicidal or homicidal thoughts.
  - Prioritize interventions to address the client's physical needs first.
- Initial interventions include the following.
  - Identifying the current problem and directing interventions for resolution
  - Taking an active, directive role with the client. Encourage active participation by the client in planning solutions and goal-setting. Qpcc
  - Helping the client to set realistic, attainable goals
- Use strategies to decrease anxiety.
  - Develop a therapeutic nurse–client relationship.
  - Remain with the client.
  - Listen and observe.
  - Make eye contact.
  - Ask questions related to the client's feelings.
  - Ask questions related to the event.
  - Demonstrate genuineness and care.
  - Communicate clearly and, if needed, with clear directives.
  - Avoid false reassurance and other nontherapeutic responses.
- Reinforce teaching about relaxation techniques.
- Identify and reinforce teaching about coping skills (assertiveness training and parenting skills).
- Assist the client with the development of the following type of action plan.
  - Short-term
  - Focused on the crisis
  - Realistic and manageable
  - Self-assessment by nurse
  - Debriefing for staff
- Critical Incident Stress Debriefing is a group approach that can be used with a group of people who have been exposed to a crisis situation.

MEDICATIONS

Administer antianxiety (alprazolam, diazepam, oxazepam) and/or antidepressant (paroxetine, bupropion, fluoxetine) medication as prescribed.

PSYCHOTHERAPEUTIC INTERVENTIONS

Primary care: Collaborate with client to identify potential problems, instruct on coping mechanisms, and assist in lifestyle changes.

Secondary care: Collaborate with client to identify interventions while in an acute crisis that promote safety.

Tertiary care: Collaborate with client to provide support during recovery from a severe crisis that includes outpatient clinics, rehabilitation centers, crisis stabilization centers, short-term residential services, and workshops.

CLIENT EDUCATION

- Services in the community can provide assistance during crises (crisis stabilization, hotlines and warm lines, mobile and peer crisis services). Qtc
- Adhere to plans for follow-up appointments.

Anger management

- Anger, a normal feeling, is an emotional response to frustration as perceived by the individual. It can be positive if there is truly an unfair or wrong situation that needs to be righted but must be expressed in a healthy manner. Anger becomes negative when it is denied, suppressed, or expressed inappropriately (by using aggressive behavior). Denied or suppressed anger can manifest as physical or psychological findings. Anger can be referred to as a secondary emotion related to another disorder (depression, unresolved grief, anxiety or unresolved PTSD).
- Aggression, whether an action or behavior, results in a verbal or physical attack. Violence is an act that is goal-directed with the intent of harming a specific person or object. Inappropriately expressed anger can become hostility or aggression. A client who is often angry and aggressive can have underlying feelings of inadequacy, insecurity, guilt, fear, and rejection.
- Despite the potential for anger and aggression among individuals who have mental illness, it is important to know that clients who have mental illness are more likely to hurt themselves than to express aggression against others.

COMORBIDITIES

- Depressive disorders
- Substance use disorders
- Bipolar disorders
- Posttraumatic stress disorder
- Alzheimer's disease
- Personality and psychotic disorders
- Individuals who are easily overwhelmed have marginal coping skills.

SECLUSION AND RESTRAINTS

Seclusion and restraint must be used only according to legal guidelines and should be the interventions of last resort after other, less restrictive options have been tried and there is a risk of harm to the client or others.

- Adhere to facility guidelines.
- Prescription from provider must include the reason for the seclusion or restraint, length of time, type of restraints, and criteria needed for removal from the secluded area or release of restraints.
- Risk of harm to client is prevented by following standards of practice and individualizing care provided.
- Client is evaluated (face to face) by health care provider, RN, or physician's assistant (PA) within one hour.
- Restrained clients are not to be left alone.
- Continuous monitoring (every 15 min) and documentation by prepared staff
- Observe for any injuries.
- Monitor for breathing or other physical difficulties.
- Anticipate need for hygiene, hydration, toileting, nutritional intake, and physical comfort.
- Assessment by RN hourly to include physiological and mental status, V/S (including pulse oximetry), review of circulatory status and skin integrity, and offering fluids
- Document all medications administered.
- If restraints have been applied, range of motion exercises are executed every two hr.
- All interactions with the client should encourage behavior that will promote release from seclusion and/or restraint.

DATA COLLECTION

RISK FACTORS

- Past history of aggression, poor impulse control, and violence
- Poor coping skills, limited support systems
- Comorbidity that leads to acts of violence (psychotic delusions; command hallucinations; violent, angry reactions with cognitive disorders)
- Living in a violent environment
- Limit-setting by the nurse within the therapeutic milieu

CLINICAL SCREENING TOOLS

- Dimensions of Anger Reactions
- Patient-Reported Outcome Measurement Information System (PROMIS)
- State-Trait Anger Scale (STAS)
- Clinical Anger Scale (CAS)

EXPECTED FINDINGS

- Hyperactivity (pacing, restlessness)
- Hypersensitivity, easily offended
- Eye contact that is intense, or no eye contact at all
- Facial expressions (frowning or grimacing)
- Body language (clenching fists, waving arms)
- Rapid breathing
- Aggressive postures (leaning forward, appearing tense)
- Verbal clues (loud, rapid talking, yelling, and shouting)
- Drug or alcohol intoxication

PATIENT-CENTERED CARE

NURSING CARE

- Provide a safe environment for the client who is aggressive, as well as for the other clients and staff on the unit.
- Follow policies of the mental health setting when working with clients who demonstrate aggression.
- Monitor for triggers or preconditions that escalate client emotions.
- Self assessment-self awareness
- Contingency management involves rewarding desired behavior, like maintaining a calm demeanor, with quantifiable rewards like handwritten notes or extended time during certain leisure activities.

STEPS TO HANDLE AGGRESSIVE BEHAVIOR

Steps to handle aggressive and/or escalating behavior in a mental health setting include the following. Qs

- Responding quickly
- Remaining calm and in control
- Encouraging the client to express feelings verbally, using therapeutic communication techniques (reflective techniques, silence, active listening)
- Allowing the client as much personal space as possible
- Maintaining eye contact and sitting or standing at the same level as the client
- Communicating with honesty, sincerity, and nonaggressive stance
- Avoiding accusatory or threatening statements
- Describing options clearly and offering choices
- Reassuring the client that staff members are present to help prevent loss of control
- Setting limits for the client
  - Tell the client calmly and directly what they must do in a particular situation, such as, "I need you to stop yelling and walk with me to the day room where we can talk."
  - Encourage the client to use physical activity, such as walking, to de-escalate anger and behaviors.
  - Inform the client of the consequences of their behavior, such as loss of privileges.
  - Use pharmacological interventions if the client does not respond to calm limit-setting.
  - Plan for four to six staff members to be available and in sight of the client as a "show of force" if appropriate.

FOLLOWING AN AGGRESSIVE/VIOLENT EPISODE

- Discuss ways for the client to keep control during the aggression cycle. Check the milieu and identify potential and actual stressors that may have contributed to the behavior.
- Encourage the client to talk about the incident and what triggered and escalated the aggression from the client's perspective.
- Participate in staff evaluation of the effectiveness of actions.
- Document the entire incident completely by including the following.
  - Behaviors leading up to, as well as those observed throughout the critical incident
  - Nursing interventions implemented, and the client's response

CLIENT DEBRIEFING

Debriefing is always completed for clients who have been placed in seclusion or restraints as soon as possible following the discontinuation of the seclusion and/or removal of restraints.

- Discussion of any misperceptions
- Display of support for client's return to unit milieu
- Identification of different approaches to prevent subsequent seclusion/restraint
- Listening to the client's point of view
- Provide guidance to the client if they believe their rights have been violated.
- Recognition of any trauma that occurred
- Adapt plan of care as needed.

MEDICATIONS

Olanzapine, ziprasidone

Classification: Atypical antipsychotics

Therapeutic intent: Olanzapine and ziprasidone are used to control aggressive and impulsive behaviors. These are used more commonly than haloperidol because of the severity of adverse effects of haloperidol.

Haloperidol

Classification: Antipsychotic agent

Therapeutic intent: Haloperidol is used to control aggressive and impulsive behavior.

NURSING ACTIONS

- Monitor for clinical findings of parkinsonian and anticholinergic adverse effects.
- Keep client hydrated, check vital signs, and test for muscle rigidity due to the risk of neuroleptic malignant syndrome.

Other medications

Other medications may be used to prevent violent behavior by treating the underlying disorder. These include antidepressants (selective serotonin reuptake inhibitors), mood stabilizers (lithium), and sedative/hypnotic medications (benzodiazepines). Qs

CLIENT EDUCATION

- Return for follow-up.
- Attend a support group.

CARE AFTER DISCHARGE

- Manage medications.
- Develop problem-solving skills.

Application Exercises

1. Place the examples of situational, maturational, and adventitious crises in the appropriate type of crises.
   A. Divorce
   B. Retirement
   C. Hurricane
   D. New job
   E. Marriage

2. A nurse is reviewing the medical records of multiple clients at a community mental health facility. Which of the following events should the nurse identify as an example of a client experiencing a maturational crisis?
   A. Rape
   B. Marriage
   C. Severe physical illness
   D. Job loss

3. A nurse in the emergency department is assisting with the care of a client who sustained minor injuries in a motor vehicle crash. The client's spouse was killed in the accident. Which of the following actions should the nurse take first?
   A. Determine if the client has thoughts of self-harm.
   B. Ask the client how the accident occurred.
   C. Assist the client in setting short-term treatment goals.
   D. Instruct the client on use of coping strategies.

4. A nurse is conducting group therapy with a group of clients. Which of the following statements made by a client is an example of aggressive communication?
   A. "I wish you would not make me angry."
   B. "I feel angry when you leave me."
   C. "It makes me angry when you interrupt me."
   D. "You'd better listen to me."

5. A nurse is caring for a client in an inpatient mental health facility who gets up from a chair and throws it across the day room. Which of the following is the priority nursing action?
   A. Encourage the client to express feelings out loud.
   B. Maintain eye contact with the client.
   C. Move the client away from others.
   D. Tell the client that the behavior is not acceptable.

Application Exercises Key

1. **SITUATIONAL:** A, D; **MATURATIONAL:** B, E; **ADVENTITIOUS:** C

   The nurse should identify that a divorce and new job are situational crises. Retirement and marriage are maturational crises. Also, a hurricane, which is a natural disaster, is an example of an adventitious crisis.

   Ⓝ *NCLEX® Connection: Psychosocial Integrity, Crisis Intervention*

2. B. **CORRECT:** Marriage is an example of a maturational crisis, which is a naturally occurring event during the lifespan. Rape is an example of an adventitious crisis. It is not a part of everyday life. Severe physical illness is an example of a situational crisis. Loss of a job is an example of a situational crisis.

   Ⓝ *NCLEX® Connection: Psychosocial Integrity, Crisis Intervention*

3. A. **CORRECT:** The greatest risk to the client experiencing a crisis is the risk of harm to themselves or others. Therefore, determining if the client has thoughts of self-harm is the action to take first. Ask the client about the accident. However, another action should be taken first. Assist the client in setting short-term goals for treatment once the acute phase of the crisis has passed. However, another action should be taken first. Instruct the client on coping strategies once the acute phase of the crisis has passed. However, another action should be taken first.

   Ⓝ *NCLEX® Connection: Psychosocial Integrity, Crisis Intervention*

4. D. **CORRECT:** This statement implies a threat and a lack of respect for another individual. The other statements are descriptions of how the client may feel and are not signs of aggression.

   Ⓝ *NCLEX® Connection: Psychosocial Integrity, Therapeutic Communication*

5. C. **CORRECT:** The behavior indicates that the client is at greatest risk for harming others. The priority action for the nurse is to move the client away from others. Encouraging the client to express feelings out loud is appropriate. However, it is not the priority action. Maintaining eye contact with the client is appropriate. However, it is not the priority action. It is appropriate to tell the client that the behavior is not acceptable. However, it is not the priority action.

   Ⓝ *NCLEX® Connection: Psychosocial Integrity, Crisis Intervention*

Active Learning Scenario

A nurse is assisting in conducting an in-service on crisis management for a group of newly licensed emergency care nurses. Use the ATI Active Learning Template: Basic Concept to complete this item.

NURSING INTERVENTIONS: Identify three interventions that can be used to assist the client who is experiencing a crisis.

Active Learning Scenario Key

Using the ATI Active Learning Template: Basic Concept

NURSING INTERVENTIONS
- Identify the current problem, and direct interventions for resolution.
- Take an active, directive role with the client.
- Help the client to set realistic, attainable goals.
- Provide for client safety.
- Initiate hospitalization to protect clients who have suicidal or homicidal thoughts.
- Prioritize interventions to address the client's physical needs first.
- Use strategies to decrease anxiety.
- Develop a therapeutic nurse-client relationship.
- Reinforce teaching about relaxation exercises.
- Reinforce teaching about coping skills.
- Administer prescribed antianxiety and/or antidepressant medications.

Ⓝ *NCLEX® Connection: Psychosocial Integrity, Crisis Intervention*

CHAPTER 25

CHAPTER 25 *Family and Community Violence*

Violence from one person toward another is a social act involving a serious abuse of power. Usually, a relatively stronger person controls or injures another, typically the least powerful person accessible to the perpetrator. This includes acts of violence that a partner commits against the other partner, adult abuse by a non-spouse or non-partner, a parent against a child, or a child against a parent.

CYCLE OF VIOLENCE

Spouse or partner violence usually follows a predictable cycle.

Tension-building phase
- The perpetrator has minor episodes of anger and can be verbally abusive and responsible for some minor physical violence (pushing, shoving).
- As tension continues to grow, both partners try to reduce it.
- The perpetrator may turn to substances, and the victim dismisses the significance of the violence.
- The vulnerable person is tense during this stage and tends to accept the blame for what is happening.

Acute battering phase
- The tension becomes too much to bear, and serious abuse takes place.
- The victim can provoke the perpetrator to reduce the unbearable tension.
- The vulnerable person can try to cover up the injury or try to get help.
- This stage is the most violent and shortest.

Honeymoon phase
- The situation is defused for a while after the violent episode.
- The perpetrator becomes loving, promises to change, and is sorry for the behavior.
- The vulnerable person wants to believe this and hopes for a change.
- Eventually, the cycle begins again.

Periods of escalation and de-escalation
- Usually continue with shorter and shorter periods of time between the two without intervention
- Emotions for the perpetrator and vulnerable person (fear or anger), increase in intensity.
- Repeated episodes of violence lead to feelings of powerlessness.

TYPES OF VIOLENCE

A nurse must prepare to deal with various types of violence and the mental health consequences.
- Violence can be directed toward a family member, stranger, or acquaintance. Or, it can come from a human-made mass-casualty incident (a terrorist attack).
- Natural disasters (hurricanes and earthquakes) can cause mental health effects comparable to those caused by human-made violence.
- Violence against a person who has a mental illness is more likely to occur when factors (poverty, transient lifestyle, or a substance use disorder) are present.
- A person who has a mental illness is no more likely to harm strangers than anyone else.
- The factor most likely to predict violence between strangers is a history of violence and criminal activity.

DATA COLLECTION

- A forensic nurse has advanced training in the collection of evidence for suspected or actual cases of sexual assault or other forms of physical abuse.
- Conduct a nursing history.
  - Provide privacy when conducting interviews about family abuse.
  - Be direct, honest, and professional.
  - Use language the client understands.
  - Be understanding and attentive.
  - Use therapeutic techniques that demonstrate understanding.
  - Use open-ended questions to elicit descriptive responses.
  - Inform the client if a referral must be made to child or adult protective services. Be sure to explain the process.

RISK FACTORS

Cultural differences can influence whether the nursing assessment data is valid, how the client responds to interventions, and the appropriateness of nursing interactions with the client. Qpcc
- **A female partner** is the vulnerable person in the majority of family violence, but the male partner can also be a vulnerable person.
- **Vulnerable persons** are at the greatest risk for violence when they try to leave the relationship.
- **Pregnancy** tends to increase the likelihood of violence by a spouse or partner. The reason for this is unclear but might be related to the added responsibility or the time that will be required to care for the infant.
- **Older adults** or other adults who are vulnerable within the home can suffer abuse because they are in poor health, exhibit disruptive behavior, or are dependent on a caregiver. The potential for violence against an older adult is highest in families where violence has already occurred. Ⓖ

FAMILY GROUPS: Violence is most common within family groups, and most is aimed at family and friends rather than strangers.

- Family violence occurs across all economic and educational backgrounds and racial and ethnic groups.
- Family violence can occur against children, spouses or partners, or vulnerable adult family members.

RISK FACTORS FOR ABUSE TOWARD A CHILD

- A child is under 4 years of age.
- A perpetrator perceives the child as being different (the child is the result of an unwanted pregnancy, is physically disabled, or has some other trait that makes them particularly vulnerable).

TYPES OF VIOLENCE

PHYSICAL VIOLENCE occurs when physical pain or harm is involved (shaken baby syndrome, strangling, striking or kicking, pushing).

SEXUAL VIOLENCE occurs when sexual contact takes place without consent, whether the vulnerable person is able to give consent or not.

EMOTIONAL VIOLENCE includes behavior that minimizes an individual's feelings of self-worth or humiliates, threatens, or intimidates a family member.

NEGLECT INCLUDES THE FAILURE TO PROVIDE THE FOLLOWING.

- Physical care, such as feeding
- Emotional care (interacting with a child, stimulation necessary for a child to develop normally)
- Education, such as enrolling a young child in school
- Necessary health or dental care

ECONOMIC ABUSE

- Failure to provide for the needs of a vulnerable person when adequate funds are available
- Unpaid bills, resulting in disconnection of gas, water, or electricity

VULNERABLE PERSON CHARACTERISTICS

- Demonstration of low self-esteem and feelings of helplessness, hopelessness, powerlessness, guilt, and shame
- Attempts to protect the perpetrator and accept responsibility for the abuse
- Possible denial of the severity of the situation and feelings of anger and terror

PERPETRATOR CHARACTERISTICS

- Possible use of threats and intimidation to control the vulnerable person
- Usually an extreme disciplinarian who believes in physical punishment
- Poor impulse control
- Perceives the victim as bad
- Violent outbursts
- Poor coping skills
- Low self-esteem

- Feelings of worthlessness
- Possible history of substance use disorder
- Difficulty assuming typical adult roles
- Likely to have experienced family violence as a child

AGE-SPECIFIC ASSESSMENTS

INFANTS

- Shaken baby syndrome: Shaking can cause intracranial hemorrhage. Monitor for respiratory distress, bulging fontanels, and an increase in head circumference. Retinal hemorrhage can be present.
- Any bruising on an infant before age 6 months is suspicious.

PRESCHOOLERS TO ADOLESCENTS

- Monitor for unusual bruising (on the abdomen, back, or buttocks). Bruising on arms and legs in these age groups is an expected finding from playing and other physical activities.
- Check the mechanism of injury, which might not be congruent with the physical appearance of the injury. Numerous bruises at different stages of healing can indicate ongoing beatings. Be suspicious of bruises or welts that resemble the shape of a belt buckle or other object.
- Monitor for burns. Burns covering "glove" or "stocking" areas of the hands or feet can indicate forced immersion into boiling water. Small, round burns can be from lit cigarettes.
- Monitor for fractures with unusual features (forearm spiral fractures), which could be a result of twisting the extremity forcefully. The presence of multiple fractures is suspicious.
- Check for human bite marks.
- Monitor for head injuries: altered level of consciousness, unequal or nonreactive pupils, and nausea or vomiting.

OLDER AND OTHER VULNERABLE ADULTS: Monitor for any bruises, lacerations, abrasions, or fractures in which the physical appearance does not match the history or mechanism of injury. Ⓖ

PATIENT-CENTERED CARE

NURSING CARE

All states have mandatory reporting laws that require nurses to report suspected child or vulnerable adult abuse; there are civil and criminal penalties for not reporting suspicions of abuse.

- Document subjective and objective data obtained during data collection.
- Provide basic care to treat injuries.
- Make appropriate referrals.
- Help client develop a safety plan, identify behaviors and situations that might trigger violence, and provide information regarding safe places to live. Qs
- Use crisis intervention techniques to help resolve family or community situations where violence has been devastating.

Interventions for community-wide or mass casualty incidents (a school shooting or gang violence)

EARLY INTERVENTION
- Make sure clients are physically and psychologically safe from harm.
- Provide psychological first aid.
- Reduce stress-related manifestations by using techniques to alleviate a panic attack.
- Provide interventions to restore rest and sleep, and connect the client to social supports and information about critical resources.
- Depending on their level of expertise and training, mental health nurses can provide assessment, consultation, therapeutic communication and support, triage, and psychological and physical care.

CRITICAL INCIDENT STRESS DEBRIEFING: This is a tertiary crisis intervention strategy that assists individuals who have experienced a traumatic event, usually involving violence (staff experiencing client violence, school children and personnel experiencing the violent death of a student, rescue workers after an earthquake) in a safe environment.
- This type of debriefing involves distinct phases: introducing the purpose of the group, discussing facts about the incident, discussing first thoughts about the incident, describing personal reactions, listing altered behaviors or physical changes since the incident, reinforcing teaching on stress management and anticipatory guidance, and providing closure to the session by affirming the participants or providing referrals as needed.
- Debriefing can take place in group meetings with a facilitator who promotes a safe environment where there can be expression of thoughts and feelings. Qᴛᴄ
- The group can choose to meet on an ongoing basis or disband after resolution of the crisis.

CLIENT EDUCATION
- Understand expected growth and development patterns for children; parenting classes can be helpful.
- Develop skills to assist with problem-solving (assertiveness training).
- Find ways to manage stress in a positive way (meditation or relaxation).
- Consider external changes that can help reduce stress (a career change or moving).

INTERPROFESSIONAL COLLABORATION
- Encourage participation in support groups.
- Use case management to coordinate community, medical, criminal justice, and social services.
- Assist with client relocation, if needed, to a safe house, shelter, a family or friend's home, or foster care.
- Discuss therapies that could be beneficial (family, individual, or partner therapy, communication courses).
- Talk with the caregivers about community agencies that could provide relief (day-care or sitter programs).

Sexual assault

Sexual assault is defined as pressured or forced sexual contact, including sexually stimulated talk or actions, inappropriate touching or intercourse, incest, human sex trafficking, female genital mutilation, and rape (forced sexual penetration). Sexual assault can be male to female, female to male, female to female, male to male. Children and vulnerable adults can also be victims of sexual assault. Sexual violence also refers to the denial of emergency contraception or measures to prevent sexually transmitted infections, organized rape during war or conflict, and sexual homicide.

Most survivors of sexual assault suffer long-term, severe emotional trauma. Rape-trauma syndrome, which is similar to posttraumatic stress disorder, can occur after a sexual assault.

RAPE

Rape is defined as nonconsensual sexual activity involving any penetration of the vagina or anus with any body part or object, or the oral penetration by a sex organ of someone else. It is a crime of violence, aggression, anger, and power.
- Types of rape include stranger, marital, date, and acquaintance. The majority of perpetrators are known to the person who is raped. Acquaintance rape and spousal (or marital) rape specify the relationship between the perpetrator and vulnerable person. Date rape is a form of acquaintance rape in which the parties agreed upon a social engagement.
- Alcohol and other substances are often associated with date or acquaintance rape (drug assisted sexual assault). These substances produce a sedative and amnesic effect on the vulnerable person.

SPECIFIC SUBSTANCES
- Gamma-hydroxybutyrate: Street names include "G" and "liquid ecstasy."
- Flunitrazepam: Street names include "roofies," "club drug," and "roachies."
- Ketamine: Street names include "black hole," "kit kat," and "special K."

DATA COLLECTION

RISK FACTORS
- There is no "typical" description of a person who is vulnerable to rape. Individuals of all ages are affected by sexual assault.
- There is no "typical" sexual assault survivor. Individuals can experience a variety of physical and emotional injuries and effects.

EXPECTED FINDINGS

Rape-trauma syndrome

Sustained and maladaptive response to a forced, violent sexual penetration against the individual's will and consent
- Initial emotional (or impact) reaction
  - An **expressed reaction** is overt and consists of emotional outbursts, including crying, laughing, hysteria, anger, and incoherence.
  - A **controlled reaction** is ambiguous. The survivor can appear calm and have blunted affect, but can also be confused, have difficulty making decisions, and feel numb.
- Following the initial emotional response, clients can experience a variety of emotional reactions, including embarrassment, a desire for revenge, guilt, anger, fear, anxiety, and denial. These reactions can persist and become sustained and maladaptive.
- A **somatic reaction** can occur later in which the client can have a variety of physical manifestations
  - Muscle tension, headaches, and sleep disturbances
  - Gastrointestinal manifestations (nausea, anorexia, diarrhea, abdominal pain)
  - Genitourinary manifestations (vaginal pain or discomfort)

Acute stress disorder

Occurs after a traumatic event (sexual assault), and manifestations are similar to posttraumatic stress disorder. In acute stress disorder manifestations appear and persist for at least 3 days and can extend to one month. Manifestations lasting longer than one month are then classified as posttraumatic stress disorder.

Posttraumatic stress disorder

Can occur beyond 1 month after the attack. Long-term psychological effects of sexual assault include the following.
- Reliving the event (flashbacks, recurrent dreams, and other intrusive thoughts about the assault)
- Increased activity (visiting friends frequently or moving residence) due to a fear that the assault will reoccur
- Hyperarousal and increased emotional responses (easily startled, anxiety, angry outbursts, difficulty falling asleep or concentrating)
- Avoidance, fears, and phobias (fear of being alone, fear of sexual encounters, avoiding triggers of the event, memory problems about the trauma, emotional numbness, guilt, and depression)
- Difficulties with daily functioning, low self-esteem, depression, sexual dysfunction, and somatic reports (headache or fatigue)

Compound rape reaction

Some survivors of rape can experience additional disorders as a result of the sexual assault.
- Mental health disorders (depression or substance use disorder)
- Physical disorders (manifestations of a prior physical illness)

Silent rape reaction

The survivor does not report or tell anyone of the sexual assault, including family, friends, or the authorities.
- Abrupt changes in relationships with partners
- Nightmares
- Increased anxiety during interview
- Marked changes in sexual behavior
- Sudden onset of phobic reactions
- No verbalization of the occurrence of sexual assault

PATIENT-CENTERED CARE

NURSING CARE

- Perform a self-assessment. It is vital that the nurse who works with the client who has been sexually assaulted be empathetic, objective, and nonjudgmental. If the nurse feels emotional about the assault due to some event or person in their own past, it can be better to allow another nurse to care for the client.
- Monitor data related to the client's level of anxiety, coping mechanisms, and available support systems. The nurse should also collect data for indications of emotional and/or physical trauma.
- Provide a private environment for an examination with a specially trained nurse-advocate, if available. A sexual assault nurse examiner (SANE) is a specially trained nurse who performs such examinations and collects forensic evidence. Qpcc
- Follow national standard protocol for the assessment, which includes client information, examination, documentation of biological and physical findings, collection of evidence, and follow-up as needed to document additional evidence.
- Provide for client safety. Let the client know they are safe. Qs
- Provide nonjudgmental and empathetic care.
- Obtain informed consent to collect data that can be used as legal evidence (photos, pelvic exam). The rape survivor has the right to refuse either a medical examination or a legal exam, which provides forensic evidence for the police.
- Treat any injuries, and document care given.
- Assist the SANE with the physical examination and the collection, documentation, and preservation of forensic evidence. Sexual assault evidence collection kits are used for collecting blood, oral swabs, hair samples, nail swabs, or scrapings, and genital, anal, or penile swabs. Document physical injuries in narrative and pictorial form, using body maps or photographs. Also document subjective data, using the client's verbatim statements.

- Support the client while legal evidence is being collected (samples of hair, skin, semen). Avoid minimizing the client's level of emotional suffering, as psychological responses can be subtle or not easily identifiable. Refrain from asking "Why" questions. Let the client know that the sexual assault is not their fault.
- Monitor for suicidal ideation.
- Administer prophylactic treatment for sexually transmitted infections as outlined by the Centers for Disease Control and Prevention. This can include prophylactic treatment of syphilis, chlamydia, gonorrhea, HIV, and hepatitis exposure. Q**pcc**
- Evaluate for pregnancy risk and provide for prevention (emergency contraception).
- Collect data regarding support systems and call the client's available personal support system (a partner or parents) if the client gives permission.
- Assist the client during the acute phase of rape-trauma syndrome to prepare for thoughts, manifestations, and emotions that can occur during the long-term phase of the syndrome.
  - Encourage the client to verbalize their story and emotions.
  - Listen and let the client talk. Use therapeutic techniques of reflection, open-ended questions, and active listening.

NURSING ACTIONS

CARE AFTER DISCHARGE
- Provide phone numbers for 24-hr hotlines for sexual assault survivors.
- Promote self-care activities. Give follow-up instructions in writing, because the client might be unable to comprehend or remember verbal instructions.
- Initiate referrals for needed resources and support services. Individual psychotherapy and group therapy can be helpful to increase coping skills and prevent long-term disability (depression or suicidal ideation).
- Schedule follow-up calls or visits at prescribed intervals after the assault.
- Emphasize importance of aftercare, as sexual assault clients historically have a poor compliance rate with follow-up visits.

1. A charge nurse is leading a peer group discussion about family and community violence. Which of the following statements by a member of the group indicates an understanding of teaching?

   A. "Children older than 5 are at greater risk for abuse."

   B. "Substance use disorder does not increase the risk for violence."

   C. "Entering an intimate relationship increases the risk for violence."

   D. "Pregnancy increases the risk for violence from a spouse or partner."

2. A nurse is preparing to collect data from an infant. Which of the following is an expected finding of shaken baby syndrome? (Select all that apply.)

   A. Sunken fontanels

   B. Respiratory distress

   C. Retinal hemorrhage

   D. Altered level of consciousness

   E. Increase in head circumference

3. A nurse is collecting data from a preschool-age child who reports abdominal pain. Which of the following findings should alert the nurse to possible abuse? (Select all that apply.)

   A. Abrasions on knees

   B. Round burn marks on forearms

   C. Mismatched clothing

   D. Abdominal rebound tenderness

   E. Areas of ecchymosis on torso

4. A nurse is preparing a community education seminar about family violence. When discussing types of violence, the nurse should include which of the following?

   A. Refusing to pay bills for a dependent, even when funds are available, is neglect.

   B. Intentionally causing someone to fall is an example of physical violence.

   C. Striking a sexual partner is an example of sexual violence.

   D. Failure to provide a stimulating environment for normal development is emotional abuse.

5. A nurse is caring for an adult client who has injuries resulting from partner violence. The client does not wish to report the violence to law enforcement authorities. Which of the following nursing actions is the highest priority?

   A. Advise the client about the location of safe houses and shelters.

   B. Encourage the client to participate in a support group for survivors of abuse.

   C. Implement case management to coordinate community and social services.

   D. Educate the client about the use of stress management techniques.

6. A community health nurse is participating in a discussion about rape with a neighborhood task force. Which of the following statements by a neighborhood citizen indicates an understanding of the teaching?

   A. "Rape is a crime of passion."

   B. "Acquaintance rape often involves alcohol."

   C. "Young adults are the typical victims of sexual assault."

   D. "The majority of rapists are unknown to the victims."

1. D. **CORRECT:** Pregnancy tends to increase the likelihood of violence from a spouse or partner. Children younger than 4 years of age are at an increased risk for abuse. Substance use disorder increases the risk for violence. Vulnerable persons are at an increased risk for violence when they try to leave the relationship.

   Ⓝ *NCLEX® Connection: Psychosocial Integrity, Crisis Intervention*

2. B, C, D, E. **CORRECT:** Respiratory distress is an expected finding of shaken baby syndrome. Retinal hemorrhage is an expected finding of shaken baby syndrome. An altered level of consciousness is an expected finding of shaken baby syndrome due to intracranial trauma or hemorrhage. An increase in head circumference is an expected finding of shaken baby syndrome. Bulging, rather than sunken, fontanels are an expected finding of shaken baby syndrome.

   Ⓝ *NCLEX® Connection: Psychosocial Integrity, Abuse or Neglect*

3. B, E. **CORRECT:** Round burn marks anywhere on the child's body can indicate cigarette burns and should alert the nurse to possible abuse. Areas of ecchymosis on the torso, back, or buttocks should alert the nurse to possible abuse. Minor injuries (abrasions) on the arms and legs are common in this age group. Mismatched clothing is consistent with the child's need for independence at this age. Abdominal rebound tenderness is a possible indication of appendicitis rather than abuse.

   Ⓝ *NCLEX® Connection: Psychosocial Integrity, Abuse or Neglect*

4. B. **CORRECT:** Physical violence occurs when physical pain or harm is directed toward another individual. Refusing to pay bills for a dependent is economic abuse, rather than neglect. Striking a sexual partner or other individual is an example of physical, rather than sexual, violence. Sexual violence occurs when sexual contact takes place without consent. Failure to provide a stimulating environment for normal development is neglect, rather than emotional abuse.

   Ⓝ *NCLEX® Connection: Psychosocial Integrity, Abuse or Neglect*

5. A. **CORRECT:** The greatest risk to this client is injury from further abuse; therefore, the priority action is to assist the client with the development of a safety plan that includes the identification of safe places to live. Encourage participation in a support group to facilitate coping. However, this is not the priority nursing action. Implement case management to assist the client with relocation or acquiring financial or other resources. However, this is not the priority nursing action. Educate the client about the use of stress management techniques to facilitate coping. However, this is not the priority nursing action.

   Ⓝ *NCLEX® Connection: Psychosocial Integrity, Abuse or Neglect*

6. B. **CORRECT:** Alcohol and other substances are often associated with date or acquaintance rape. Rape is a crime of violence, aggression, anger, and power. Individuals of all ages are affected by sexual assault and can be male or female. The majority of perpetrators are known to the vulnerable persons.

   Ⓝ *NCLEX® Connection: Psychosocial Integrity, Abuse or Neglect*

References

Alegria, M., NeMoyer, A., Bague, I., Wang, Y., & Alvarez, K. (2018, September). Social determinants of mental health: Where we are and where we need to go. *Current Psychiatry Reports, 20*(95). https://doi.org/10.1007/s11920-018-0969-9

American Psychiatric Association. (2022). *Diagnostic and statistical manual of mental disorders* (5th ed.).

ATI Nursing. (2022). *Engage fundamentals* (1st ed.).

ATI Nursing. (2022). *Engage mental health* (1st ed.).

Berman, A., Snyder, S. & Frandsen, G. (2021). *Kozier & Erb's Fundamentals of nursing: Concepts, process, and practice* (11th ed.) e-book. Pearson.

Burchum, J. R. & Rosenthal, L. D. (2022). *Lehne's pharmacology for nursing care* (11th ed.). Elsevier.

Centers for Disease Control and Prevention. (2021). *Suicide.* https://www.cdc.gov/suicide/index.html

Columbia Suicide Severity Rating Scale (C-SSRS). (2014). *Substance abuse and mental health services administration (SAMHSA).* https://www.samhsa.gov/resource/dbhis/columbia-suicide-severity-rating-scale-c-ssrs

Halter, M. J. (2022). *Varcarolis' foundations of psychiatric mental health nursing: A clinical approach* (9th ed.). Elsevier.

Kikuchi, T., Maeda, K., Suzuki, M., Hirose, T., Futamura, T., & McQuade, R. D. (2021). Discovery research and development history of the dopamine D2 receptor partial agonists, aripiprazole and brexpiprazole. *Neuropsychopharmacology Reports, 41*(2), 134-143.

Mayo Clinic. (2019). *Tricyclic antidepressants and tetracyclic antidepressants.* https://www.mayoclinic.org.diseases-conditions/depression/in-depth/antidepressants/art-20046983

Mayo Clinic. (2020). *Schizophrenia.* https://www.mayoclinic.org/diseases-conditions/schizophrenia/symptoms-causes/syc-20354443

National Institute of Mental Health. (2021). *Frequently asked questions about suicide.* https://www.nimh.nih.gov/sites/default/files/documents/health/publications/suicide-faq/suicide-faq.pdf

Potter, P.A., Perry, A. G., Stockert, P. A. & Hall, A.M. (2021). *Fundamentals of nursing* (10th ed.). Elsevier.

Townsend, M. C., & Morgan K. I. (2020). *Essentials of psychiatric mental health nursing: Concept of care in evidence-based practice* (8th ed.). F.A. Davis.

Vallerand, A. H., & Sanoski, C. A. (2021). *Davis's drug guide for nurses* (17th ed). F.A. Davis.

STUDENT NAME _____

CONCEPT_____ REVIEW MODULE CHAPTER_____

Related Content

(E.G., DELEGATION, LEVELS OF PREVENTION, ADVANCE DIRECTIVES)

Underlying Principles

Nursing Interventions

WHO? WHEN? WHY? HOW?

STUDENT NAME _____

PROCEDURE NAME _____ REVIEW MODULE CHAPTER_____

Description of Procedure

Indications

CONSIDERATIONS

Nursing Interventions (pre, intra, post)

Interpretation of Findings

Client Education

Potential Complications

Nursing Interventions

Growth and Development

STUDENT NAME _____

DEVELOPMENTAL STAGE _____   REVIEW MODULE CHAPTER_____

EXPECTED GROWTH AND DEVELOPMENT

Physical Development	Cognitive Development	Psychosocial Development	Age-Appropriate Activities

Health Promotion

Immunizations	Health Screening	Nutrition	Injury Prevention

STUDENT NAME _____

MEDICATION _____ REVIEW MODULE CHAPTER_____

CATEGORY CLASS_____

PURPOSE OF MEDICATION

Expected Pharmacological Action

Therapeutic Use

Complications

Medication Administration

Contraindications/Precautions

Nursing Interventions

Interactions

Client Education

Evaluation of Medication Effectiveness

STUDENT NAME _____

SKILL NAME_____ REVIEW MODULE CHAPTER_____

Description of Skill

Indications

CONSIDERATIONS

Nursing Interventions (pre, intra, post)

Outcomes/Evaluation

Client Education

Potential Complications

Nursing Interventions

System Disorder

STUDENT NAME _____

DISORDER/DISEASE PROCESS _____ REVIEW MODULE CHAPTER_____

Alterations in Health (Diagnosis)

Pathophysiology Related to Client Problem

Health Promotion and Disease Prevention

ASSESSMENT

Risk Factors

Expected Findings

Laboratory Tests

Diagnostic Procedures

SAFETY CONSIDERATIONS

PATIENT-CENTERED CARE

Nursing Care

Medications

Client Education

Therapeutic Procedures

Interprofessional Care

Complications

STUDENT NAME _____

PROCEDURE NAME _____ REVIEW MODULE CHAPTER_____

Description of Procedure

Indications

CONSIDERATIONS

Nursing Interventions (pre, intra, post)

Outcomes/Evaluation

Client Education

Potential Complications

Nursing Interventions

STUDENT NAME _____

CONCEPT ANALYSIS_____

Defining Characteristics

Antecedents

(WHAT MUST OCCUR/BE IN PLACE FOR
CONCEPT TO EXIST/FUNCTION PROPERLY)

Negative Consequences

(RESULTS FROM IMPAIRED ANTECEDENT —
COMPLETE WITH FACULTY ASSISTANCE)

Related Concepts

(REVIEW LIST OF CONCEPTS AND IDENTIFY, WHICH
CAN BE AFFECTED BY THE STATUS OF THIS CONCEPT
— COMPLETE WITH FACULTY ASSISTANCE)

Exemplars